Living with Lung Cancer

My Journey

by Thomas E Cappiello

© 2012 by Thomas E Cappiello
First Edition – September 2012

Front Cover Photo: Thomas and Yoko Cappiello. Photo courtesy Paula Kennedy Photography. Copyright 2007 by Paula Kennedy Photography.

ISBN
978-1-77097-703-7 (Hardcover)
978-1-77097-704-4 (Paperback)
978-1-77097-705-1 (eBook)

All rights reserved.

No part of this publication may be reproduced in any form, or by any means, electronic or mechanical, including photocopying, recording, or any information browsing, storage, or retrieval system, without permission in writing from the publisher.

Published by:

FriesenPress

Suite 300 – 852 Fort Street
Victoria, BC, Canada V8W 1H8

www.friesenpress.com

Distributed to the trade by The Ingram Book Company

Library of Congress Cataloging-in-Publication-Data
Cappiello, Thomas
Living with Lung Cancer — My Journey and Other Essays on Life by Thomas Cappiello — First Edition P. CM
   1. Cancer 2. Survivor 2. Biography, 3. Cancer — Popular works
   Includes bibliographical references and index

A portion of the proceeds from the sale of this book will be donated to support lung cancer research and early detection. For more information about advocating for lung cancer or to contact Thomas Cappiello visit www.livingwithlungcancermyjourney.com

Table of Contents

Introduction.. vii

A Note to Readers.. ix

Part I — 2007.. 1

Part II — 2008.. 45

Part III — 2009... 81

Part IV — 2010... 95

Part V — 2011... 161

Epilogue — A Second Chance at Life 211

Acknowledgements 215

This book is dedicated to my loving wife, Yoko, and my three beautiful daughters, Paula, June and Jessica.

You are my life and my reason for living.

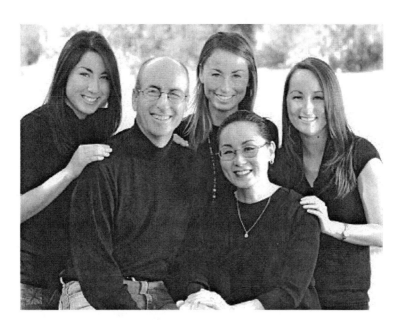

Photo courtesy of Paula Kennedy Photography

Introduction

On October 5 2007 at the age of 52, I was diagnosed with Stage IIIA locally-advanced adenocarcinoma (Non-Small Cell Lung Cancer). This book is a compendium of online diary entries and essays over the past five years. Initially my purpose in writing was for emotional therapy. I was in shock. I thought my diagnosis was terminal. I suddenly felt an urgent need to record the events of my life for future generations.

I believed I was facing an early death. I was afraid of what might come next for me and my family. There were things I wanted to say to my children that I might never have a chance to say. I wanted to leave a written account of my life and my life-lessons so that I would not be quickly forgotten.

From the day of my diagnosis, routine life was put on indefinite hold. All our plans for the future were suspended. I entered a period of uncertainty and emotional turmoil. The most immediate question I had after being diagnosed was what comes next? How does this disease progress and how long do I have to live?

These writings and essays were meant to be a way for my children to remember me and my un-born grandchildren to know me. Eventually, I realized I would be a survivor and death was not imminent. I began to live again with renewed purpose and energy. I realized how short life can be and there was so much more I wanted to accomplish. I got busy living life again.

I thought my experience could give other lung cancer patients and their caregivers hope. After finishing a year of treatments, I embarked on writing a column called "Living with Cancer" for Sun Newspapers in 2008.

Since being diagnosed with lung cancer I learned that it is among the deadliest of cancers, accounting for a third of all cancer deaths. People think that smoking is a prerequisite for developing lung cancer. That isn't true. Anyone with lungs can develop the disease. Lung cancer among "never smokers" is the sixth leading cause of all cancer deaths. The fact is we don't know why some people develop lung cancer and others do not. More research is needed and it is why I am a lung cancer advocate.

I hope this book and the telling of my story will give newly diagnosed lung cancer patients an idea of what life is like living with cancer and what comes next.

The journey is different for everyone, but my hope is that, no matter the stage of your disease, my story will inspire you to fight hard and live another day. I survived late stage lung cancer. So can you.

Every minute of life is a precious gift from God. There is no time to waste.

Thomas E. Cappiello
February 19, 2012

A Note to Readers

When speaking about lung cancer mortality, morbidity, incidence, funding, and survivorship, I have tried to be as accurate as I can be using sources I believe to be reliable. The reader should be warned, however, that statistics used in this book were correct to the best of my knowledge at the time of my diary entries or when my columns were originally published. To be consistent with respect to the timeline of when I was writing, I have not attempted to update these numbers, which have changed somewhat in the intervening years.

I have not written this book as a lung cancer specialist. I am not a physician. I am a patient and survivor/advocate. My descriptions of medical procedures and my understanding of the biology of cancer are as a layman. I believe that my entries are fundamentally correct, but to the extent they are not, only I am to blame.

Part I — 2007

October 27, 2007 — My Background

I live in Punta Gorda, a beautiful little coastal town on the West Coast of Florida, where I work as a financial advisor. I have been married to my kind-hearted and beautiful wife Yoko for 26 years. We have three lovely daughters. Paula is a 25-year old first grade teacher living in Bakersfield California; June, 22, lives in Honolulu, Hawaii, and works for the Kahala Hotel and Resorts. My youngest daughter Jessica is 19 living in Tallahassee and attending Florida State University. I love them all with all my heart. I never say that enough. Now that I have been diagnosed with a terminal disease, I try and tell them every day.

I was born in Stamford, Connecticut on October 16 1955 and raised there until about the age of seven. I have a brother and three sisters, all of a similar upbringing. Everyone in my immediate family is alive and well, except my father, Frank, who passed away in 2002 from multiple causes. I really miss my Dad, but at least I had him to turn to well into my married life. It makes me sad to think I might not be there for my daughters the way my Dad was there for me.

My brother had prostate cancer last year, which was treated by removing the prostate. My father also had prostate cancer, but doctors treated his less radically with seed radiation. My 84-year-old mother has had breast cancer, twice now, and is being successfully treated with radiation. Cancer in my family is a new phenomenon.

My family (except my sister Peggy, who was yet to be born) left Stamford in 1962 and moved to Syracuse, New York where my father worked as a manufacturer's rep. My sister Peggy became a part of the family in 1966. In the summer of '66 my father's job took him to Pennsylvania, so we moved again. I have a few childhood memories of Stamford, more of Syracuse, but most are clearly of Horsham, PA which is where I really say I am "from" when people ask.

When we moved to Pennsylvania my Mom got involved with hosting exchange students from the University of Pennsylvania. I remember one year she invited a Japanese couple to our home for Thanksgiving. The woman wore a kimono for the occasion. They were the first Japanese I ever met. My mother's involvement with hosting international students had a huge impact on my life.

In high school I decided I wanted to go abroad for a year and experience another culture. I heard about the Rotary Student Exchange Program through friends and decided to apply. Little did I realize how this decision would impact the rest of my life. At the end of my junior year in high school I was selected to represent my Rotary district as an exchange student to Izumiotsu City, Japan (near Osaka) for one year. It meant having to give up graduating with my friends and attending high school for an extra year. I graduated from high school in 1974.

Had I not gone to Japan as an exchange student, I might never have taken up cigarettes. The Japanese kids I hung out with all smoked and I would go with them after school to the "Spot Five" coffeehouse, where you could listen to music, drink coffee, smoke and talk. Unfortunately for me, smoking cigarettes became a life long addiction.

In hindsight leaving the familiar behind and going to Japan was one of the best decisions I ever made. That year in Japan opened my eyes to the world and changed my life forever. I learned to speak Japanese (something I still work on). I attended The George Washington University so I could continue studying Japanese. I took Japanese at Georgetown University and, after graduating in 1978, found a job in Japan.

My first employer was a well known company, Nissho Iwai, headquartered in Tokyo. They were a large general trading company. My job in the PR department was to produce an English language magazine, English language annual report, represent the company to the foreign press, etc. I worked for Nissho Iwai for four years and I must say that it was a formative experience. There are lots of stories but the most important was that working there led to meeting my wife, Yoko, one night. We dated for three years before we were married in May of 1981. We had our first child, Paula, in March of 1982.

The summer after Paula was born we decided that Yoko needed to learn to speak English and I needed to get a graduate degree in business. So in July of 1982 we moved back to the US. I enrolled in the two-year MBA program at Penn State.

In January of 1984, having finished all my graduate school class work, Yoko and I packed up and moved to California so that I could begin work for the (now defunct) accounting firm, Arthur Andersen & Co. Paula was not even 2 years old. We lived in Contra Costa County in San Francisco's East Bay. My job was to help organize Arthur Andersen's marketing effort aimed at selling audit and tax services to Japanese companies investing abroad. My daughter June was born — aptly — in June 1985, just before we moved into our first house.

My growing family lived in California for three years — until October of 1986, when I was reassigned to work for Andersen in Tokyo. My daughter Jessica was born in Tokyo in 1988, at the height of the Japanese foreign investment boom. I stayed with Andersen in Tokyo until 1994. By that time, the Japanese investment boom had ended and it was not clear what more I could do for the firm. My career path was uncertain and I began looking for new opportunities.

In May of 1994 I quit Arthur Andersen to begin a software start-up, which I ran as founder and CEO for three years. In 1997, I began looking for buyers of the business and sent Yoko and the girls back to the States. They landed in Punta Gorda Florida, where my parents were retired, in July of 1997. After selling the assets of the company to a European buyer, I followed Yoko and the girls to Punta Gorda in the spring of 1998 and sat for the license to be a stockbroker in October 1998. I began my second career as a financial advisor in 1999.

I love to golf, ski, ride horses, read history, write, eat out and travel. I have an interest in music and modern art and recently purchased my first collector artwork. With enough time my ambitions would include writing a screenplay, collecting art and learning to paint, attending plays and concerts and working on other outlets for my creativity. Now that I am facing a shorter life expectancy, I am trying to get it all done at once.

I was raised as a Catholic and believe in God, but for me, religion is about your personal beliefs. Yoko converted to Catholicism before we were married. Her parents were both Buddhist and Shinto. I would say that Yoko and I are both more spiritual than we are religious.

So now you know, in a nutshell, my life story and how a Japanese-speaking financial advisor ends up in Punta Gorda, Florida learning to live with cancer.

November 2, 2007 — The Diagnosis

I developed a cough this past summer that I could not shake. The funny thing is that, after years of trying, I finally quit smoking in February 2007 using a prescription drug called varenicline (Chantix®). Over time, I became more concerned about the cough because, no matter what I did, it would not go away. I thought it might have been allergies or maybe dust or mold in the office. The cough seemed worse at work than at home, so I was convinced it had to be allergies. I tried all kinds of over-the-counter allergy medications but nothing seemed to help.

I finally made an appointment to see my primary care doctor for my annual physical. My doctor ordered chest x-rays and I went for the x-ray the same day as my appointment. That was October 3, 2007. The next morning I received an ominous phone call from my doctor, saying he wanted to see me immediately.

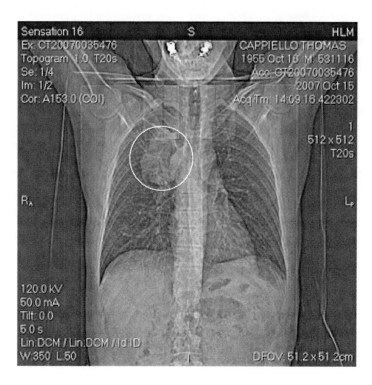

A chest x-ray plainly shows a large tumor in the right upper lobe

At our meeting, my physician said he discovered a shadow in my chest x-ray that was "disturbing". He wanted me to immediately go (that day) for a CT scan and biopsy. One of the things I learned about cancer is that, once discovered, you are in hurry-up mode to get a handle on it as quickly as possible. My doctor arranged for me to go to a local imaging center the next day, where I had the CT scan followed by a CT guided needle biopsy. On Friday October 5, I was confirmed, according to the pathology, to have adenocarcinoma — a form of Non-Small Cell Lung Cancer (NSCLC).

At its largest point the tumor measured about 9 cm in size — about the size of baseball. My physician advised me that he would refer me to a medical oncologist and that it would be necessary to have a PET scan to see if the cancer has spread. We had the PET scan done that day, and I was set for an appointment with my oncologist, Scott Lunin (herein referred to as Dr. Scott) with Florida Cancer Specialists and Research Institute.

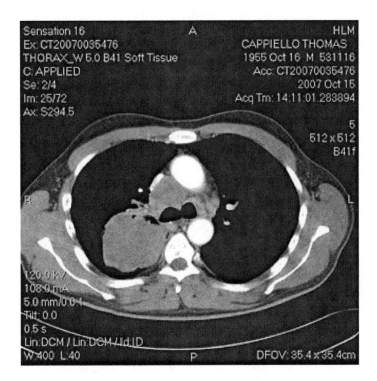

When Yoko and I met with Dr. Scott he explained my diagnosis was Stage IIIA Non-Small Cell Lung Cancer. The primary tumor was quite large and localized in one area of my lung. There is no sign of cancer anywhere else. Had the cancer spread (say to my left lung), I would be considered Stage IIIB or even Stage IV if the cancer spread (metastasized) outside the lung and there were tumors elsewhere. Dr. Scott explained that there is some involvement in the hilar lymph node (a lymph node in the middle of the chest) which is also concerning. He recommended that I begin chemotherapy treatment right away using two drugs, Cisplatin and Taxol. We talked a lot about the side effects of these drugs and their toxicity, but whatever the side effects, it was better than the alternative.

Dr. Scott said he did not believe that surgery would be possible until the tumor was smaller. (The tumor is in my right upper lung posterior, adjacent to the mediastinum. See x-ray.) Had the tumor been smaller, surgery followed by chemotherapy would be the best option for long-term survival, which in the world of cancer is considered to be five years, but unfortunately, like most lung cancer patients diagnosed today, surgery is not an option. Most lung cancers aren't spotted until they are locally advanced or already metastasized, which is the reason that lung cancer mortality is 85 percent within five years. A tumor in the lungs can't be felt because there are no nerve endings in the lungs. Lung cancer also generally does not cause symptoms (such as a cough) until it is well developed. Stage I and II lung cancer patients are often treated with surgery. For Stage III and IV, surgery is usually more problematic.

Dr. Scott said he was not a surgeon but he thought surgery would be out of the question until we could "shrink" the tumor with chemo. He immediately arranged for me to meet with Dr. Lary Robinson at The Moffitt Cancer Center, in Tampa. Dr. Scott said Dr. Robinson was one of the premier thoracic surgeons in the country. If Dr. Robinson would not surgically remove the tumor, no one would. We needed to know whether the tumor could be surgically removed or not in order to make a decision on the course of treatment.

We met with Dr Robinson on October 15. His view was, not only was I not a candidate for surgery, I would not be a candidate for surgery anytime in the future either. He pointed out that the tumor was impinging on the superior vena cava, a major vein that returns blood from the head (See CT-scan). If the tumor were not immediately dealt with, there was a chance that I could have a stroke or have some other major complication and cancer would be the least of my problems.

Dr. Robinson believed that the best course of treatment would be to immediately start combined chemotherapy and radiation. Radiation, I was told, is not something you want to do if you are going to have surgery because radiation tends to result in scar tissue forming and "blurs" the lines between the tumor and good tissues and makes "getting it all" more difficult. Also, tissue that is radiated does not heal as well and that makes future surgery more difficult.

Radiation, on the other hand, tends to be more effective when combined with chemotherapy. It is settled then. Surgery is out of the question, at least for the time being.

I had my first chemo treatment on October 18, with a plan to follow-up with radiation the following week. Dr. Scott set me up with a radiation oncologist (herein named Dr. Dave) who I met years ago on the golf course. (He is a scratch golfer, which gives me confidence.) I am now undergoing a regimen of chemo once a week and radiation every day. The course of treatment will continue for seven weeks of chemo and 35 days (5 days a week) of radiation. The chemo is supposed to sensitize the tumor; the radiation will do the heavy lifting

November 3, 2007 — Chemotherapy Treatment

I began chemotherapy treatments on Thursday, October 18. The current round is planned to be eight weeks of chemotherapy, to coincide with seven weeks (35 treatments) of radiation. My plan is to have the treatments every Friday. That way, if I am feeling some side effects, I would have the weekend to recover before going back to work the following Monday.

I am to get a variety of drugs each week as follows:

- Aloxi (an anti-nausea drug)

- Decadron (a steroid, anti-inflammatory immunosuppressant; helps the anti-nausea effects of Aloxi)

- Tagamet (for acid reflux)

- Benadryl (an antihistamine given to prevent a potential allergic reaction to Taxol)

- Taxol (a cancer (antineoplastic) medication; it interferes with the growth of cancer cells and slows their growth and spread in the body.)

- Potassium

- Magnesium

- Lasix (a diuretic given to help reduce the amount of water in the body. They work by acting on the kidneys to increase the flow of urine.)

- Mannitol (to induce urination and prevent excess body water)
- Cisplatin (a platinum-based drug known to interfere with the growth and spread of cancer cells)

The bags of potassium and magnesium are to counteract the effects the Cisplatin has on reducing these chemicals in the body and to help "flush" the kidneys, which can be damaged by the drug.

It takes about six hours to be fed the drugs via IV. I show up at the cancer treatment center around nine in the morning right after my radiation treatment. They first take blood for testing and, if everything looks OK, I am taken to the treatment room to receive the IV. They have a solarium and some comfortable lazy-boy type chairs. A nurse will hook me up with an IV and set the drugs, which are numbered, on a stand with a pump. I can read a book and listen to my i-pod while receiving treatment. I am generally finished around 3 P.M.

I have been surprised at how little I have had in the way of side effects from treatment so far. I was expecting much worse. On the first round of chemo I vomited only one time and that was "not much" because Yoko was feeding me like a bird. I seem to get tired easily, but not sleepy.

After the first treatment we went to Houston to visit with my Mom and my sister Peggy. I was tired and slept during the day, but I was not the exhausted tired that I was expecting. I seem to get feverish once in a while, but if I take a short nap, I seem to recover pretty well.

I have always been able to sleep, but since the diagnosis I sleep for an hour or two and wake up, look at the clock, and try and fall asleep again. I am not sure if this is the drugs or something psychological. Maybe it is the stress and worry about what is going to happen. When I do sleep something always seems to wake me. Most nights it is heartburn or acid reflux. Other nights it is Yoko who can't sleep and wakes me up. Last night it was a rash.

I had an allergic reaction to something and I broke out in an itchy rash across my chest. The rash was like a poison ivy rash in appearance; I showed it to Dr. Scott and he brought in a colleague to look at it. He had the "I've never seen this before" look in his eyes.

He and his associate agreed that the rash appeared to be a drug reaction, but it would be hard to know which drug. He tried to see if I had eaten something unusual or if Yoko was washing the clothes with a different detergent. I told Dr. Scott I suspect that the rash is a delayed reaction; that perhaps some of the drugs in the chemo cocktail masked the reaction but wore off over time. His colleague thought it could be the Taxol. The rash developed over several days and got bad only last night. After today's infusion the rash almost completely disappeared. In fact, there was a noticeable improvement WHILE chemo was being given, which seems to support my theory.

It is 3 A.M. and I am up writing because I can't sleep. The steroids energize me and keep me up at night. I had enough acid reflux tonight to cause a violent vomiting episode. Of course I feel better afterward! Hopefully this vomiting will be a one-time event.

They say I have to maintain my weight and I am actually eating better than I did before my diagnosis. I would say before all this began I weighed 155 stark naked. In fact, I was developing love handles and I thought I was getting too heavy in the wrong places. So before I was diagnosed, I was frequently skipping breakfast and often lunch and just eating one full meal a day. In hindsight, I now realize that my "dieting" may have been a loss of appetite associated with the tumor.

I am now making it a point to eat three meals (or more) a day. When I went for my annual physical, I weighed 149 with all my clothes on. (They weigh you these days with shoes on, so who knows what your actual weight is…it depends on whether you have beach sandals on that day or leather wingtips!) After three weeks of treatment I weighed in at 148 (fully clothed). The radiation people began to lecture me about how important that I NOT lose weight! (Next week I am going with the wingtips!) My goal is to get back to 150 fully clothed.

I have not had to deal with many other side effects. They say the Cisplatin can affect your kidneys, so I am drinking water frequently. I was starting to get some back pain, but that has gone away and so has my cough (mostly) so that is good news. I have not lost any more hair than when I started, so no one knows I am being treated for cancer — no one will notice if I lose more on my head; if I lose my eyebrows, that is another story and I will have to think about what do, since I do not want the world to know about this yet. It is a matter of time, I suppose.

November 4, 2007 — Who Should Know I Have Lung Cancer?

When I first learned I had lung cancer I was devastated. This kind of a diagnosis and the prognosis feels like a death sentence. The thing is I did not commit any crime. Smoking was an addiction. I could not quit — try (many times) as I did. I wish I had never started. I don't mind being a hypocrite in telling my kids not to smoke.

The first thing I had to deal with after the diagnosis was "who to tell." My wife and I talked about this a lot. I am somewhat well known in this little community because of my civic involvement, the fact that I am marketing my name and watching over the financial investments of hundreds of households. I don't know what my long-term prospects are. Luckily, a few years ago I took on a young man as a partner in my practice. I say luckily because, not only is he doing a good job in helping me sell our services, he is in a position to easily take over my practice and serve my existing clients if I die or am disabled.

The uncertainty of what happens next makes deciding who to tell all the more difficult. How sick am I going to become? Will I be able to work during treatment? If treatment does not work, what happens next? How will the disease progress? At what point will I not be able to effectively take care of business? What should I tell people who are thinking of becoming my client? Am I morally obligated to tell them I have cancer? Should I tell my clients why I am not in the office on Fridays (because of chemo) or should I let them continue to believe that I am out golfing?

My wife and I concluded together that it is best that we keep this matter private and tell people on a "needs to know" basis for now. The only people who know about this at the moment, outside of my family, are my partner, my branch and complex manager, and the southern regional manager. If I am going to be missing a lot of work, I needed my partner to know so that he can cover. The office manager should know why I am not in the office and

I need the branch manager to know, because he is my profit and loss reporting relationship. The complex manager should know because he is the one that hired me and I had immediate questions about my employment agreement. I have not told anyone else in the office.

As far as having to reveal my condition to my clients, I have concluded I would rather not for now. Frankly I don't know what good it would do to tell them. While my long term prognosis is not very good as a general statistical measure, (only a 15% chance of living five or more years) the fact of the matter is that the statistics reflect a population that is significantly older than me. And older people would likely have other complicating conditions.

I do not have diabetes, COPD or other lung disease or breathing problems, etc. This helps me. On the other hand, I am Stage IIIA, I have lymph node involvement and the tumor is inoperable. That works against me.

Realistically, I think I have a good one-year chance for survival and only a fair five-year chance of survival. There is no need to rush out and tell the world. I have time. In six months, I will know better. If at that time the prognosis is worst, I will have come up with some sort of transition/succession plan. My main concern is that, while I am being treated, my clients are properly served.

So far the side effects have not given me away...but that may not last. The other problem I have is I keep running into people I know at the doctor's office. So far I am batting 1,000 in terms of seeing people I know. The first week I went to see Dr. Scott, I ran into one of my former clients. He is 93 years-old and did not recognize me. The next time I was at Dr. Scott's office, I saw people I know from Rotary. They did not see me hiding in a magazine.

Today I did not see anyone I know, but of course, if anyone knows my name it does not help when the nurse comes into the waiting room and calls out Cappiello. Not only does everyone in the waiting room now know who you are, but if they recognize your name, it won't be long before they tell someone. I think they ought to use numbers instead of names — like the deli — when it's your turn to be served in a cancer clinic.

Anyway, keeping a secret in a small town is hard. It is going to come out eventually and I will have to deal with it. Bottom line — if I had AIDS or any other disease — I would not feel obligated to disclose the fact to my clients. I don't know with any more certainty today when I am going to die than I did a month ago. It could be tomorrow or it could be in 5 or 10 years from now.

I have concluded that I wish to lead my life as normally as I can. I am not going to go around acting like I am going to die soon. I will plan for the worst, to be prudent, but I am going to act like anyone with a normal life expectancy and then see what develops. As far as getting new clients, I think the same holds. I am selling the team concept and a process. My process is not dependent on me alone, so I am less concerned.

What about family? It goes without saying that I have to tell my children and immediate family. We made that decision after we got the diagnosis. I am keeping this blog for them. I hope they will read the entries and comment or make suggestions, as I intend to be very open and plain in my writings. I also hope you who are reading this will quit smoking. It is not too late.

What about friends? Well I can't tell my friends who live in the immediate area. If I do that I might as well just tell the whole community. So I am electing NOT to tell my friends. I hope they will understand my reasoning. My first obligation is to take care of my family. I am the family breadwinner and I am in a business that is difficult in the best of circumstances. I don't want my clients to panic and "bail" on me because I may not be around. That does not help them or me. And I don't want to be stuck in neutral, unable to get new clients because of concerns over my health.

So for now, the best answer for me and my family is to keep this a private matter and just go on as we have. If my condition deteriorates, I will have to reconsider what to do, but as long as I can function normally, I don't see a need to make a general announcement. Having said that, I would LOVE to tell my brothers in Rotary, my friends at the free clinic, my golfing friends and especially my friends who are still smoking, that I have lung cancer. I'll say now that I am sorry to have had to keep this from you, though I am sure you will understand.

Monday, November 5, 2007 — Radiation Treatment

On Thursday night I had to pack the office for our move to a new location. I was tired and I must have overdone it. When I came home my ankles were swollen and I had a rash. Of course, any little thing and Yoko is bugging me to call the doctor. Instead I called my sister Jane, who is a nurse. It is not unusual to have swelling in the ankles during chemo. According to Dr Scott, fluids can accumulate in the extremities and "leak out." Anyway, I asked Dr. Scott about this and he did not seem too concerned. Sure enough, then next morning the swelling was gone, despite all the physical activity this weekend.

Friday I had chemo. Friday night Yoko, Jessie and I ate together. Actually, Yoko is keeping the daily details of what I am eating. Here was Friday evening's menu: pounded, paper thin veal (breaded and fried), spaghetti in marinara sauce, mixed salad and bread. For dessert we had homemade apple pie, oranges, ice cream and coffee. I went to bed early, at 10 PM, and I was up at 2 AM Saturday morning, spewing all that good food! Oh well.

Simultaneously with chemo, I am getting radiation treatment. Apparently, radiation in combination with chemo is more effective in killing cancer cells than either treatment alone. I have been going for radiation every morning for the past two weeks and I will be going for another five weeks.

Each day I show up for treatment at 8:50 AM. My chest area has been marked with some small tattoos so that they can line me up in the machine with precision. Then the machine starts humming and the staff who positioned me leaves the room and closes the vault door behind. The machine moves around me...each time positioning for the next blast of rays. The rays are being aimed at the cancerous tumor from six positions. It takes the machine a minute to assume each position and shoot the rays (30 — 50 second blasts); the whole treatment process takes no more than 10 minutes. I asked this morning and was told I am getting two grays per treatment. If that is true, then I am getting 70 grays because I am scheduled for 35 treatments.

The treatment has been totally painless and I am not suffering any ill effects. Radiation is going to lead to scaring of these organ tissues and I am told I may find it somewhat harder to breathe or swallow for a while. To date I have had no discomfort, but the effect of the treatment is cumulative. I am starting to feel some stiffness in my chest when I swallow, but at this point it is hardly worth mentioning. The key, in any event, is to eat and maintain your weight. So far that has not been a problem.

I worked a full day today and feel fine. No cough, no rash, no itching, no swollen ankles, no acid indigestion, no bowel trouble, and no (additional) loss of hair...in short I feel fit as a fiddle and more optimistic that I can beat the odds.

Now that I am facing something that may ultimately lead to my demise, it occurred to me that it would be a very good time to begin thinking about religion and the life hereafter. On the way home from golf, I passed the San Antonio Catholic church near my home, and stopped to see if the sign in front tells when they hear confession. Nothing was posted, so I guess I will have to call. It has been so long since I went to confession; I may have to make a special appointment!

We have a full week coming up: On Wednesday I am hosting 100 people for a private art show. Thursday evening I have a seminar with about 30 people coming. Friday is chemo day and the beginning of our hosting a weekend Rotary guest... Hopefully the treadmill I ordered is going to show up this week. Then I can REALLY start running.

November 6, 2007 — Leaving a Family Legacy

Since being diagnosed with lung cancer I have begun to think about my legacy and what I am going to leave behind for my children and grandchildren. Of course, I am hoping to beat the cancer and live long enough to enjoy the next stage of my life. I am looking forward to watching Paula, June and Jessie get married and start families themselves. This is the culmination of everything Yoko and I have worked for. But if I am not there, what have I left behind and what will they have to remember me by? What will be my legacy?

My uncle Sam has a log-cabin retreat with 100 or so acres in a beautiful spot in upstate New York. I have often told Yoko that I would love to leave land to my family — a family estate. My dream would be to have a beautiful 100-acre working horse farm. This would be a place to retire — perhaps in New Mexico or someplace like that, and then could be passed on from generation to generation. My wife is so practical, however. Yoko says: "well, who is going to pay for the upkeep? What about the taxes and insurance? And my response is, "uh… it's just a dream… I haven't worked out the details yet." But she's right… and now I may not have the time to realize my dream — which, until now I figured was 15 years or so away. Lately, I have begun to think that art, rather than land, might be a more practical asset to pass on to future generations.

I am not an artist, but I love art. Before I learned about my cancer, the plan was to begin traveling. We made it to Hawaii in late July for a family summer vacation. Yoko and I spent a lot of time visiting art galleries around Waikiki. A few weeks later we were off to Fort Lauderdale for a weekend getaway. We went to visit an old college friend who lives in Miami Beach. He is a criminal tax defense lawyer and lives on an exclusive private island off of South Beach. My friend collects art and has some easily recognizable pieces. One I noticed in his living room was a piece by Joan Miró, the Spanish artist. (Miró has a very distinctive style and once you know what he does, he is as easily recognizable as Jackson Pollack.) In fact, he was a student of Picasso's and you can see Picasso's influence in his work.

The following day Yoko and I were touring Las Olas Blvd in Fort Lauderdale just browsing art galleries, when we happened into the New River Gallery. They ALSO had a Miró original…this time with a price tag. (Yikes!) Yoko and I had a long talk with the gallery consultant, who explained how they help people become collectors …and that is when I began to think it would make a great hobby and perhaps a good investment. I decided to study the idea a little more.

For Labor Day, Yoko and I went with friends to New Mexico, spending a lot of the time in Santa Fe looking at art. A few weeks later, we went to New York City to see friends. While we were there we went to The Museum of Modern Art, where we saw more Miró. We also visited the Metropolitan Museum, where we saw many of the great 21st century artists, including Miró.

I had been bumping into Joan Miró everywhere. Perhaps it was a sign. I had never really considered buying anything like this. After my lung cancer diagnosis, it dawned on me that this might be a great legacy and gift to my children and future generations.

A few weeks ago, in the midst of all this news about cancer, I decided to bite the bullet. I am now the proud owner of Joan Mirós Pygmies Sous La Lune (etching and aquatint) Number 17 of 50 original productions.

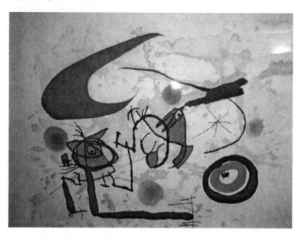

November 7, 2007 — The Beauty of Crazy Ideas and Experiments

The curator of the New River Fine Art Gallery in Fort Lauderdale came to Punta Gorda to be the speaker at a private art show we held tonight for my clients and guests. Featured artists included Picasso, Miró, Royo, Jamali, and Dali.

Yoko and I both thought the event was a success. We had about 70 guests, most of whom were either clients or potential clients. The event was planned as a "thank you" for my clients. It had been planned well before I found out about my cancer. We were nervous that I would not be physically able to hold the event (because of the effects of treatment) but as things turned out, I felt fine. In fact, we went out to dinner afterward and had a very enjoyable evening. I am feeling none the worse despite having left the house this morning at 8:30 AM and not returning until 10 P.M. If I am supposed to be run down and fatigued, I sure don't feel it! I had a full meal — Caesar salad, fillet mignon, spinach and risotto, followed by cheesecake and a cappuccino. I don't think anyone would guess I am going on my 3rd week of chemo and radiation. We are now going to plan an even "bigger" show for next year — God willing.

Of course, none of our guests knows anything about my diagnosis. Cancer, nevertheless, comes up frequently in conversation. Several of my clients, including a husband and wife, were diagnosed with cancer in the last few weeks. He has prostate cancer and she has breast cancer. Another guest had a "family emergency" and had to leave the event early because his brother-in-law took a turn for the worse. (His bother-in-law discovered he had colon cancer six months ago.) Someone else I was talking to today just had surgery to remove a tumor and could not attend the event. And, of course, there is another client of mine who could not make tonight's event because he has been diagnosed with cancer of the esophagus and is undergoing intensive chemo treatment. How I would love to tell these people that I know what they are going through!

A few people thought I was crazy for buying the Miró abstract; but most people — after they heard Larry's presentation, explaining how Miró created the piece — a "color wash and aquatint etching" — and the amount of time it took (one year) could understand. My "Pygmies" was created toward the end of Miró's life in 1972 — 1973, when he was experimenting with aquatint.

And what's the moral of today's story? I guess there is a certain inspiration we can take from someone like Miró, who kept experimenting with new things, even at the age of 90. I want to keep trying new things too. It was experimenting that came up with some of these (seemingly) crazy treatments for cancer — injecting platinum into patients; radiating them with photons. Great ideas sometime start with seemingly crazy notions. Maybe that's why Miró makes sense to me.

November 8, 2007 — Emotional Ups and Downs

Tomorrow is the anniversary of my third week since beginning treatment. Tomorrow will be my fourth chemo treatment (which generally is taking six hours each time). After tomorrow's treatment I will be more than half way home. I have had 14 radiation treatments (28 grays); I will be half way done with radiation when I hit treatment 18 next Thursday.

I believe the treatment is working. I do not cough at all anymore; a month ago I could not stop coughing. I am not vomiting as I did before treatment began. (I got sick twice last week, after chemo, but since then I have been taking Aciphex on a daily basis and I have not gotten ill at all.) I was very arthritic before treatment began. If I sat in my recliner for an hour, I was struggling to stand up because I was stiff. The stiffness has gone away. Apparently the steroids they give me in chemo helps but I believe the tumor was producing chemicals that made me arthritic.

All these symptoms going away suggest to me that the tumor is shrinking and that the treatment is working. So I am feeling optimistic. My cousin Sammy called today asking after me and I told him that, if anyone is positioned to beat the odds, it is me. I am younger than most people who are diagnosed with lung cancer. I have no complicating health issues. We caught it at stage IIIA, not early, but not TOO late; the cancer has NOT metastasized, as far as we know, and I am tolerating the current treatment extremely well. Unless I told them, no one could tell by looking at me that I am being treated for cancer. In fact, I would venture to say I am in better shape than when I was diagnosed. I am feeling optimistic.

What about my mental state? Anyone that knows me knows how emotional I am. I lost it one night a few years ago, when I was speaking in front of a large gathering at a Rotary dinner. I had been president of the Peace River Rotary club that year (the year Hurricane Charley blew down my house). As club president, I was the one who was able to hand out $40,000 in checks to hurricane victims and help families get back on their feet. As I was recounting all the good things we did as a Rotary club that year, I got all choked up and could not finish what I had to say. The thing I most clearly remember about that night, however, was the president of our local hospital, coming up to me afterward and saying, "don't worry about it; it takes a pretty big man to cry in front of all these people!"

I am even more emotional these days. One of my favorite musicals is *South Pacific*; I can hardly watch it because I get so choked up with emotion. I see so much of my own life in the story, which is about inter-racial relations, love, conflict and overcoming bigotry. These days, almost anything can set me off. I get choked up watching the sunset. I get choked up reading some of these entries out loud. I am not sad or depressed — just more emotional (than normal).

This weekend we have a Frenchman coming to stay with us for three days beginning Saturday afternoon. He is a Rotary Group Study Exchange (GSE) student we agreed to host. We have to figure out how to entertain him and I am wondering what we are going to do. Perhaps we will go golfing or take a boat trip down the Peace River. If his name is Emile, I'm toast.

November 10, 2007 — Putting Steroids to Good Use

I am not sure what steroids do for cancer treatment, but I do know they get me pretty hyped up! According to the nurses I asked, it is not uncommon for people being treated with chemo and steroids to become energized and sleepless. It's a common complaint. So here I am again at 2 AM, unable to sleep and raring to go like the energizer bunny. I knew this was coming. I should have hooked the new treadmill up to a generator. I could have lit the city of Punta Gorda tonight.

After dinner I did a little work on my blog — called my Mom to see if she was getting my e-mail to her OK — and then sat down to watch a movie, Godfather III, which I have seen a million times but Yoko did not really remember. I love most Mafia movies (*The Godfather Trilogy*, *The Sopranos*, etc.) I think part of the reason is that I can relate to the idea of family as it is portrayed in these movies. Michael Corleone is a tragic character and so is his father, Vito. They are heavily influenced by Sicilian culture; they did not start out as bad guys; they were trying to take care of their families and bring "justice" to the world. They come to realize that the world is corrupt and that there is no justice and really no difference between powerful politicians (who are corrupt) and powerful "criminals." Michael and Vito Corleone see themselves as people aspiring to power and getting what is rightfully theirs for their family. They don't see themselves as criminals. I see them as heroic (albeit ruthless and immoral) but tragic characters. They are brave and willing to do things that most other people would never consider doing. You have to admire their bravery and their ability to commit outrageous acts to further their goals. They have certain wisdom about people and the world.

Anyway, at the end of Godfather III, Michael Corleone has achieved his life's ambitions. He has extricated his family from criminal activity, he has won back the love of his wife, he has watched his son begin a career in the "legitimate world", he has confessed his sins, and he has relinquished his responsibilities as head of the family. He has abandoned ambition. But the one thing he was trying to do his whole life — protect his family — is lost. His innocent daughter is murdered in the end by a bullet meant for him.

What makes Godfather III tragic is that Michael is NOT killed — his daughter is the one to die. HE lives to be an old man. That is a tragedy because his life's work — all he had achieved — was in vain. Without his daughter living a full and happy life, HIS life had no meaning. He would not allow her to be with the man she loved. Symbolically, his success in stopping the relationship kills her and kills his family. He dies unhappy and alone. For Michael Corleone, it would have been better had the bullet killed him.

At one point in the movie — when Michael tries to convince Kay he is not a bad man, he says "I would give my soul for my family." I think that sums up his thinking and motivation. Nothing is too much for his family. My father was that way. So am I. I think most fathers (Italian or not) feel that way, which is why these Mafia movies appeal more to men than they do to women.

Women have different sensibilities than men, but I am not sure I have been able to teach my girls about men. They just think I am not like them. I guess they will find out soon enough. Just remember girls, women and men are NOTHING alike! And double that if the woman is Japanese and the man is an American!

I am reading "Team of Rivals" which Mom gave me for my birthday. Most of what we know about people in the Lincoln administration, which is what the book is about, comes from the letters and diaries that they wrote. They did not have TV, the Internet, i-pods and other modern distractions. They read (sometimes the same book over and over till it was memorized) and they wrote a lot. That is how we learn about their mind set and what they were thinking. And that is why people in that era could recite whole passages of books or poetry...just like I know most of the lines from *Casablanca* and other movies I have seen or the words of hundreds of songs I have heard over and over again.

Thankfully we have the writings of historic figures in diaries and letters where they would express their inner self. We still have to interpret what they say, but we have a much better insight into their personalities. I would venture to say we know more about historic figures of the 17th, 18th century and 19th century than others because they wrote about their lives extensively and they wrote well. When I was growing up, diaries were "encouraged" but it was work. I did keep a diary for much of the year I went to Japan in high school. Now I wished I had kept a diary my whole life.

There are so many stories I want to tell. Maybe I can remember enough to tell some. But as time goes on, months and years are lost to memory. When we were in New Mexico my college friends were recounting the time they came to visit Yoko and me at Penn State. They remembered the trip as if it were yesterday, yet I don't even remember them coming to visit us there...See what I mean? Maybe if I had kept a diary, I would remember. Yoko's theory — like all Japanese — is that taking lots of photos it is a way of jogging the memory and keeping precious moments alive.

What I have discovered by writing every day is that there is a lot of stuff that goes on in everyday life. If you start to record it and reflect upon it, you may end up discovering that your everyday life has something going on that is interesting, funny or fun. An interesting life can pass you by if you don't stop and look at the life you have and really appreciate it. Count your blessings. Realize that there are always people around you with worse problems and you will be satisfied with what you have. If you get depressed or down about your life or the circumstances you find yourself in, watch an episode of COPS on TV. My father use to say, "The grass is always greener on the other side of the hill." You should realize that the other side of the hill might be a cliff. Be happy for the green grass you live in.

People are never just satisfied with what they have. They always want more. They can't get more soon enough and once they have it, it is never enough. The moral is that if you seek material wealth in this world and never give anything back, you are never going to be truly happy or satisfied.

Families should be more like the Cratchets — not Scrooge — in a Christmas Carol; cheerful in whatever circumstances you find yourself and happy with the caring and love you share in one another. We help one another and look out for each other. We are all invalids, like Tiny Tim, in some way. No one is perfect. In families you try to look past imperfections.

Since I have been writing every day, I have begun to reflect on my life to date and realize what a blessed and unusual life I have had. I am grateful to be able to go through something like this with a wife and three daughters, a mother, and other family who care about me. I am working and insured. We are not going to be bankrupted by all this; we can afford the best care. I live at a time when fantastic technology can extend my life well beyond what it might otherwise be. I have traveled all over the world; I have met Presidents and Prime Ministers, and many persons of note. If I am going to be killed by something at an early age, I would rather like to have time to be prepared and prepare the people around me. I am not happy about getting lung cancer, but all in all, it could be worse.

A friend of mine named Dennis, also 52, was killed this year in a freak car accident. It was a shock because it was so sudden. I hope I live another 20 years, but if not, I am grateful that I now can really appreciate whatever time I may have left. The last years may be the best and most meaningful of my life. This really would have been tragic if it had happened 10 years ago. My kids are now adults or very nearly there and Yoko will have the three girls to count on. I am glad for that. My family will be OK. Now I am hoping to accomplish a lot in the time I have left. I feel I have wasted a LOT of time and I hope, in my final years, I can teach my children not to do the same.

My legacy is my children and what I have taught them. They and their children are the ones who can change the world for the better. They should think about that — how their life and work will change the world.

Paula has found teaching. What a great profession! She loves it and she can have a huge impact on many people for the rest of their lives. It is not just a job to pay the bills. Perhaps SHE should start a diary about the kids she is teaching and how she copes with everyday life. Maybe she would get a lot out of this kind of self-reflection about what she is doing and why.

June is just getting started and trying to survive on her own. She is living in Hawaii and working in one of the most beautiful places in the world. June is so smart and talented. She needs to realize that she can do anything she wants to do in any field. I have high hopes and aspirations for June. Whatever she does I know she will have a big impact.

Jessie is just starting college and I tell her that she should keep an open mind and take classes and get involved in lots of different things. She is hard working, extremely people smart, and beautiful. If she can fend off the boys long enough and balance her social life with academics and intellectual pursuits, she too will find something that she loves. The key is keeping an open mind and trying lots of different things and meeting lots of different people.

Everyone tells us that we have great kids. We really do. Mostly I credit Yoko for raising the girls. I was working and never around much to have an impact. I DO want to take credit for going to Japan to find Yoko and bringing her back here. I will also take credit for the tough love side of raising our kids. Yoko could never say no. But I can't imagine what my life would have been like without Yoko or "my girls." I am truly a blessed man.

November 14, 2007 — Cancer is everywhere!

I had an appointment with a couple who had been at my seminar last week. We talked for three hours. It took me an hour into the conversation to learn that the woman had been diagnosed with brain cancer in 2002. They removed most (not all) of the tumor and she is now on medication, but she has survived for more than five years with this diagnosis. The cancer did not metastasize and she appears to be doing well. Once she got cancer, she went on disability right away and will be collecting disability for the rest of her life. As a person receiving disability from Social Security, she is able to receive Medicare as well.

No sooner did this first prospect leave than my next appointment called to cancel. She was in severe pain. She explained that she is being treated for breast cancer and that the disease had metastasized. The pain, she says, comes and goes. When the pain comes it is debilitating. I asked her where she is being treated. Turns out she is getting chemo at the same place I go.

Not a day goes by that I don't talk with someone who has cancer, is a cancer "survivor", or has a friend or relative with cancer. As long as I can remember we have talked about cancer, but I don't ever remember a time where it has hit this close to home with so much frequency. Maybe it is just the place where I live (the oldest county by average age in the United States) or maybe it's just me. It feels like an epidemic. Everywhere I turn there is another cancer victim.

Tomorrow I will have my 19th radiation treatment and my fifth chemo treatment. I spent the entire week doing the things I always do. Tonight I had another investment seminar and got home at 9 PM.

Last week I learned that Dr Scott has been reading my blog prior to our appointment and was able to tell me how I was feeling as I walked into the examine room. I would like this blog to be a test to see if he does it again:

Dr. Scott, I feel fine. I have a rash on my skin you should check out that I think is from the radiation. Also Yoko has a rash on both her arms and wants to know if that could be caused by contamination from me. Other than that, I have no complaints. I think you'll find I weigh the same 149 pounds. My lungs are clear. No joint pain. I have no cough. You can feel my neck and shoulders but I don't think you will find anything. (What are you looking for anyway?) I'm betting that my blood work will remain within the normal range. I am less tired than I was in week one and two. I did not come home to take a nap or alter my normal schedule in any way. I don't think by looking at me you would have any idea I am being treated for cancer.

I DO have a few questions this week; if I am tolerating the treatment this well, why would we not increase the dosage of Taxol and Cisplatin? Wouldn't we be better off to be more aggressive now? Is the low dosage approach in consideration of keeping me working or my desire not to let people know? Does that kind of thing influence your thinking when you decide dosage? (Note to readers: I later learned that doctors who follow "evidenced based medicine" don't decide dosage on a whim. They follow clinically tested dosing regimens as a "standard of care.")

My second question is what thoughts you have with regard to a continuing regimen once we do the re-staging. Last week you intimated that you would plan to continue treatments after re staging. What drugs do you have in mind? Would the next stage of chemo be similar to the current stage (i.e. once a week for six hours)? I feel I need to keep after this thing. My question is what comes next.

November 20, 2007 — Next Steps

I have to say Dr. Scott has been extraordinary. I had a nosebleed yesterday, and he was immediately on top of it. I let him know I had a nosebleed by e-mail (Yoko insisted) and he immediately replied back to me on how I should take care of this and the possible cause. It may be from the chemo or it could just as well be from my "prying" fingers. (I am stuffy and it has been very dry around here lately.) Dr. Scott later called me just to check on me. It is obvious he is paying attention and cares about the patients he is treating. It gives me confidence that I am getting the best care from a doctor who is truly concerned about my well-being. I hope my clients feel about me the same way I feel about Dr. Scott. He's terrific.

I find it extraordinary that Dr. Scott is calling me at all hours of the day and night to check on me or to discuss my case. It would be one thing for him to call if I were sick and looking for help; but I have really been quite fine — if not improved — throughout treatment so far. I have only two chemo treatments to go and

14 radiation treatments. I weighed in today at 151 pounds, so I GAINED weight this week. Dr. Scott has been very pro-active in treating me and thinking about what can or should be done.

One of the things I asked about and Dr. Scott is giving serious consideration to is what the "next steps" should be. Assuming surgery is out — what is the next best course of action? To his credit, Dr. Scott is reaching out to colleagues he respects in the medical community to consult on my case. It is very reassuring to know that he is using the resources at his disposal to get the best minds available weighing in on my case.

This morning he called me on my cell, because he was about to talk to Dr Frank Fossella at The MD Anderson Cancer Center in Houston. Dr Fossella is a leading thoracic surgeon who specializes in lung cancer only. I could not join the conversation because I was sitting with clients myself. Dr. Scott wanted me to hear this from the horse's mouth to gain a better appreciation of the complexity of the issues and biology involved.

My nature is to simplify and estimate in order to find solutions to complex problems. (I learned this trick in college from a lifelong friend, Luther Liggett.) I'm not good with complexity.

At 8:30 tonight Dr. Scott called to relay the gist of the conversation with Dr. Fossella. We talked until about 9:15. This memorializes what Dr. Scott and I discussed. If I have it wrong or am misinterpreting or misstating what was said, Dr. Scott can straighten me out when I see him on Friday.

The real question I have is — assuming this thing progresses as it "normally does" — what would be the next step? The answer is that there is no "normal progression." Dr. Scott tried to explain how complex the biology is when it comes to cancer. That you can have two people — subjected to identical treatments — and end up with polar opposite results. In one case the cancer (tumor) melts away; in another case it does not or worse, it grows or metastasizes during treatment. These are opposite results and no one can say with any certainty which outcome I might have. No one knows why you get two polar opposite results — because they don't fully understand the cell biology of cancer. What we are left with, therefore, is a trial by error approach — to see what works. Try this — try that...

The next step, though, is to re-stage, that is, check what stage my cancer is at now, after my treatment. The idea of re-staging is to measure the success or failure of a given treatment regimen. Until we re-measure, there is no saying what next steps should be.

I explained to Dr. Scott that, in my job, I deal primarily with probability and outcome. I don't know what the stock market is going to do on any given day, but I DO know that I have a one in three chance of having a positive year, and that the odds of having positive returns improve with time. My concern about "next steps" has as much to do with planning my life for the next three months as it does with anything else.

I explained that my thinking about this is that, even if we don't know what the outcome will be, we should know a range of outcomes from most likely to least likely. The question I ask is whether the tumor "melting away" is like winning the lottery? Sure it could happen, but I am not betting my financial future on having that lucky ticket. Now if he tells me that chemotherapy and radiation results in the tumors melting away 50% of the time, that would be encouraging, but I have gathered just from the survivor evidence (high morbidity) that that is certainly NOT the case. I think Dr. Scott conceded that the "melting away" outcome is possible but not a likely outcome.

Can we get enough shrinkage that surgery becomes an option? Again, I think the honest answer is "probably not." We are not ruling surgery out entirely and we are certainly going to ask again and re-confirm that surgery is definitely off the table. I think, at this point, that the likelihood of surgery happening is remote to none. The tumor is simply too "involved" with the central chest for this to be a realistic hope. But it does not hurt to ask one more time.

Where does that leave us? Radiation can only go on so long before it does more harm than good. After receiving 70 grays, this tumor is cooked and I confirmed that we would not look to any further radiation on the tumor beyond the definitive treatment we are currently doing. To do more risks harming good tissues in the lung, heart, etc.

If you eliminate radiation and surgery, all that is left is chemo. Dr. Scott and I agree that we will probably need to look at some continuing chemo regimen. I think that even if the tumor "melted away" we would still be looking at further chemo.

The chemo I am currently getting is to treat the locally advanced tumor and is a "definitive" chemo radiation treatment, meaning that this is currently considered the most effective treatment for trying to control this particular lung cancer. We have to understand that "most effective" does not necessarily mean "effective." That is to say, it may or may not work.

Once we complete the definitive treatment, which is really aimed at the lung tumor itself, we should probably look at a continuing treatment regimen that is optimized for systemic treatment of cancer. That is to say, to try and stop the cancer from spreading or growing elsewhere. Dr. Scott is considering a number of drugs and regimens. Dr Fossella thinks it would be reasonable to perhaps provide me with the same treatment that I might be provided post-operatively were I to have surgery. The problem Dr. Scott has with this is the "minimal" improvement in longevity — perhaps 5% — for the effort and risk of side effects. Whatever next steps we take will have to consider the risks to my general health. That is what will make this a hard decision.

At the end of the conversation, my takeaway was that continuing treatment by chemo starting in February is the most likely scenario. We are likely to look at a different mix of drugs, focusing more on the systemic treatment. Whatever the case, the treatments early next year will likely involve more side effects, lower blood counts, the need for shots to counteract the chemo, and other measures, and will not likely be as "kind" as this first round of chemo has turned out to be. I may be looking at weekly (or more frequent) treatments.

November 28, 2007 — "Curb Your Enthusiasm"

In my world these days, no news is good news. Nothing exciting has happened in the last few days and there is nothing to report. I got a call from Dr. Scott, who read a prior blog and called because he wanted to know what color my phlegm is. (The answer is clear). The conversation went like this: "Hey Tom, it's Scott again. What color is your phlegm?" I'm telling you...this doctor is on top of things! I will see Dr. Scott tomorrow for our final chemo treatment.

Radiation goes on as usual. I am counting down the days to the end of these treatments because it is starting to get uncomfortable. I had my normal breakfast this morning and a late lunch at Amimoto, where Yoko works. I did not have much of an appetite this evening. Yoko made clam chowder. I had that and watermelon for dinner. By the end of the day I am very tired and just want to go home and rest. Last night I was in bed at 9:30 PM and slept until 8 AM. I felt better this morning but I still have a low level of energy. I worked until 5:30 P.M. and came home.

I am starting to feel guilty about being as well as I am right now. I've got all the readers of my blog upset and praying for me...and I appreciate the prayers, but suggest they may want to save some for if and when I REALLY need them.

I was saying to Yoko tonight that I feel like Larry David, who stars in the HBO sitcom "Curb Your Enthusiasm." In one episode Larry "discovers" that telling people "my mother died" is the perfect excuse to get out of anything he doesn't want to do. Someone calls up and invites him to a party; he doesn't want to go so he says, "I can't...my mother died." No one blames him for staying home. In the episode Larry uses "my mother died" to get anything he wants or to get out of doing anything he does not want to do.

Along the same lines, "I have been diagnosed with inoperable lung cancer" should be a great get out of jail free card. The best part of this is I am not in declining health at this stage, so now would be the time to play the cancer card. I will have to think about how to use it!

Aunt Sue called to say hello to Yoko. Yoko was very happy to get the call and just chat. She also got a call from my high school friend, Linda and from my sister. It's good you are calling Yoko. She can use the support. Yoko and my girls are the ones who are going to need help and support. Not me. I feel terrible that they have to go through this.

Yoko wants me to keep my daily writing honest and not to write for an audience. I am worried about wearing my heart on my sleeve for the world to see. I don't want to embarrass my mother, so I have avoided swear words and profanity. To be honest, I would have chosen different language for my "Don't Screw with me...I have Cancer" T-shirt.

I must say it is very nice to get comments and notes from my sisters and my children; at this stage, it appears, I can say or do no wrong. No one disagrees with anything I have to say! Hmmmm.... Cue the tuba.

November 29, 2007 — Thoughts about Cancer Research

Today was my seventh (and hopefully last) chemo treatment. I left the house at the usual time...8:35 A.M., had radiation at 8:50 A.M. I was taking chemo by 9:15 A.M. I got home at 3:30 P.M. and took a two-hour nap. I feel fine. I am starting to wonder if they put any drugs in those bags! Actually, I got pretty sleepy from the Benadryl and slept for a large part of the infusion time.

The treatment room was busy and I could not get my usual chair in the sun, so I sat in a chair near the nurses. The room was freezing and, even covered in a blanket, I was cold. Those nurses are wonderful. I can't imagine doing what they do all day everyday... but I must say they are very professional and competent and treat you like you were the first patient they ever had.

Not being able to find a chair made me think of all the people being treated for cancer. You have to wonder where the incentive is to find a cure. This is very big business. I never really realized just how big a business cancer is — I might have intellectually known it was big, but I never really saw it on a day to day basis as I do now. The sheer number of cases out there is amazing. The incentive to find a cure I suppose is the dollars that will be saved in the health care system. We need a cure rather than treatments.

In the meantime, oncologists have a business model that just won't quit. They don't have to go out and do seminars and scratch and claw to find new business like I do; it comes waltzing in the front door every day. Dr. Scott's waiting room is bigger than my entire office in Punta Gorda!

Anyway, I was thinking about all this and, after watching the presidential debates last night, it dawned on me that our national priorities are really screwed up. The National Institutes of Health has a $28 billion budget. Over $2.3 billion is going to AIDS research; all cancer together is about $4.3 billion. Lung cancer, which kills more people than all other cancers combined, has the lowest funding. Try these statistics on for size: The 5 year survival rate for breast cancer it is 87%; for prostate cancer it is about 99%; for colon cancer it is about 64%; for lung cancer the 5-year survival rate is 15%. (For Stage III lung cancer, which is what I have, it is just 5 %.)

If you do the math, and assume a US population approaching 300 million, that would mean there are about 226,000 cases of lung cancer and 229,000 cases of breast cancer that will be diagnosed this year. Of the breast cancer cases, 1% or 24,000 cases a year will succumb to the disease within 5 years. For lung cancer, almost 190,000 of those people will die within 5 years. We spent $781 million on breast cancer research in 2007, $380 million on prostate cancer, $270 million on colon cancer, and $297 million on lung cancer, which kills more people than all the others COMBINED. Good God. Why don't we put more money into fighting lung cancer?

You want to hear the kicker that adds insult to injury? The Federal government collects nearly $8 billion a year (39 cents a pack) on cigarette sales. I think current smokers and former smokers need to demand that the sin tax the federal government collects be used for cancer research. What do you think? I would spend most of those dollars first to find ways of safely detecting lung cancer early — perhaps finding a genetic marker or blood marker (like the PSA for prostate)? (Editor's Note: In late 2010, the National Lung Screening Trial conclusively showed that CT screening for lung cancer of those at high risk saves lives from the disease). If lung cancer were simply found early, survival rates would jump significantly.

November 29, 2007 — The Key to Cancer Survival and Life Lessons

I recently read something really interesting. Because cancer grows geometrically, you can think of it like algae on a pond that doubles in size every day. Eventually the cancer takes over the organ it has invaded. The earlier you catch it the better off you are. The article was saying that if the algae were on a pond, and the algae doubled in size every day to cover the pond in 30 days, how long before the pond was covered would you want to detect and treat the cancer? Counting backward, half the pond is covered on day 29. One quarter of the pond is covered on day 28. Most people only find the cancer (allegorically) 3 or 4 days before the pond is covered. That is why early detection and prompt treatment are at the heart of treating the disease successfully. Early detection is what mainly accounts for the differences in survival rates between the various cancers.

What is OBVIOUSLY needed is a better way of detecting lung cancer. X-ray is simply too crude a tool and NOT nearly good enough. I had an X-ray 2 years ago and nothing was detected. Had I had another X-ray in 2006 we might have found the tumor earlier. Yoko's mother (she NEVER smoked) had lung cancer. She survived 15 years because her cancer was found at a stage where she could have surgery. They were able to remove a section of her lung and she lived 15 years, until she was 77 years old.

Anyway, sitting there in the chemo treatment room, filled to the brim with cancer patients, I started thinking about what we lung cancer patients need to do. We need some national leadership on this. Write to your congressman and senators. Send them this article and demand they take action. Lung cancer patients need to get better organized and compete for available funding. People have asked me why lung cancer is not better organized. The answer is that, when you are dying, political advocacy is not high on the agenda! We need to get a national spokesman, like Peter Jennings or Dana Reeves. Oh wait…damn… they're not available. If I get well, I'll do what I can.

Your view of life changes when you know your time on earth may be limited. It changes your perspective and suddenly you want to go out and do good deeds. I think this is natural and is often reflected in the inspirational talks by people diagnosed with a terminal disease. Jimmy Valvano and Randy Pausch are two people who come to mind.

The message is always the same: love and care for your family, help others, and do something to make the world a better place before you leave it. I think most people living their daily life don't recognize all the capacity we have to love, do good and change the world for the better. I thought the Jimmy V comments said it all when he said, if you laugh, think, and cry once a day, you are living a full life. By those standards, I am living a very full life these days!

For me, keeping this diary has been a great way of documenting what I am doing and feeling each day and reflecting on how I am leading my life and using my time. I would like to set a good example for my children, in the time I have, to show them all the possibilities that life offers.

Speaking of opportunities, I found a cruise aboard the brand new Queen Victoria that would leave from England and take you around the world for only $22k per person (drinks and excursion fares separate). Aside from the fare, the only problem is the 106 days you need to make the trip. I wonder if I have enough time.

December 5, 2007 — Chemo One More Time

Well, I thought I was done with chemo for now, but after seeing my radiology oncologist yesterday, he recommended that I have one more chemo session. The radiation is the main element of the treatment that is killing the tumor; the chemo sensitizes the tumor so that the radiation does a better job. Anyway, I have a scheduled chemo session for Friday morning...and then, hopefully, that will be it for the Christmas season.

My last radiation session is next Tuesday...the same day the Federal Reserve will decide whether to cut interest rates. Tuesday should be a good day!

The difficulty eating I am currently experiencing should abate after radiation ends. In the meantime, I have been reduced to eating things that are easily broken up and swallowed, like tuna salad, soups, rice dishes, etc. Last night Yoko made stuffed green bell peppers. They are bell peppers stuffed with rice and mixed with ground beef and tomato sauce. She tops them with melted cheese. Delicious! Of course, when she serves the food, I want to swallow the whole thing in one gulp, but I am forced to eat it slowly in tiny bites, which is very frustrating when you are hungry and the food in front of you smells and looks so great!

I saw an advertisement in the newspaper the other day that was quoting Abraham Lincoln as saying, "It is not the number of years in a life that counts…it is the life in the years" or something along those lines. Having reflected a lot lately about my life, I really cannot complain. Of course, I would like to do more, but I am also sure that even if I were 80 years old I would be saying the same thing. Anyway, relative to vastness of infinite time, what is the difference between 50 and 80 years…not much.

The real waste is when young people don't get the opportunity to have a life. On the web I am reading about a 15-year-old girl with Stage IV lung cancer fighting for her life. Reading about her plight brings tears to my eyes and makes me determined to advocate for lung cancer research. No. She NEVER smoked.

I watched a movie last night called *Alpha Dog*, with Bruce Willis. It is apparently a true story about a screwed up teenage drug-dealer kidnapping and then killing the innocent younger brother of an addict who owes him money. The kid that was murdered was 15 years old. The amount of money that was owed was $1,200. The story takes place in 2003. As I watched all I could think of was how selfish people are. Everyone is looking out for number one… and the innocent die as a result. What a waste.

Then in today's newspaper there was a story about an environmentalist who decided to have an abortion and then elected to be sterilized so that her "carbon impact" would be reduced. My question is, for whom is she saving the world? If everyone followed this lady's philosophy, there would be no one around to enjoy the clean lakes and clear blue sky. Like the newspaper editorial said, I never read a good book by a polar bear.

Tonight Yoko and I are attending our last evening Rotary Dinner of the year. It should be a good time. As we do every year, club members will be bringing gifts (one for a boy and one for a girl) to donate to a local charity called "For the Love of Kids." I was also glad to learn that my Rotary District provided $55,000 to outfit the Children's Hospital in Fort Myers with a playroom for kids with cancer. To me, THAT is what the Christmas season is all about. God Bless Rotarians!

December 8, 2007 — Chemo is finished at Last!

It took a little longer than usual to finish yesterday's treatment. I did not get home from chemo until 3:40 PM. That makes for a long day of doing nothing. I was going to read and work on my laptop during the chemo infusion, but after the first bag of Benadryl I fell asleep. I drifted in and out of sleep the whole time, while listening to music on my i-pod. Jessie made me a 250-song play list of the music she listens to. It is really pretty good. I could never embrace rap music at all, but it looks like the young people today are getting back to music with melody and harmony. I'm sure Jessie would be surprised to learn that I like a lot of the music she listens to.

Speaking of music, Yoko had the TV on yesterday morning and there was a show about one of the icons of my generation, Bobby Dylan. God, he is/was an awful singer. I don't know how or why he became so popular. I said this to Yoko and she agreed; but then she reminded me that we bought the Miró abstract! Talent and beauty is in the eye of the beholder, I guess.

What a great idea for my mother to send airline tickets to Paula and June so they could come home this Christmas! We are so excited to be able to see all our girls together! I have been thinking about what to get everyone. I am having a hard time coming up with ideas.

I got my hair cut very short this week to cover up the fact that I have begun to lose my hair (more quickly than usual). A golfing buddy — who has no idea I have cancer — kept making comments about how skinny I am and how I looked like I was on chemo — ha ha ha. All I could say was, "Watch it...you'd feel terrible if it turned out I actually had cancer!" Of course, everyone was chuckling. It was all I could do not to tear off my shirt and show them my tattoos. I wanted to say, "I AM undergoing chemo and radiation. It's no joke, asshole! Even though it hurts to swing and my blood count is well below normal, even in my weakened state I still play better golf than any of you!" I resisted the temptation of course...but I would really like to tell my friends about my diagnosis.

After golf came the big challenge — eating lunch. I piled on the easy to eat bake beans, potato salad and slaw and got one hamburger. It still took me an hour to eat. (To give you an idea of how slow this is, one of my friends had the same side dishes PLUS two hamburgers and a hot dog...and went back for seconds. Another finished his first plate of food before I even sat down! They both finished two plates before I had even eaten half of mine.) The hardest part is not grimacing as you swallow. At least at home I can moan as I eat! Anyway, I was able to finish what I had taken before the event was over. Tonight we have the company Christmas party. It is a sit down dinner. I guess we will go...but I sure hope they serve macaroni and cheese!

All this has made me think that perhaps it is some sort of omen that my last chemo took place on December 7th — Pearl Harbor Day. The first battle is over but the fight has just begun. Take that you rat bastard cancer cells!

December 11, 2007 — The Genie is out of the Bottle!

Today was my last day of radiation. The nurses wanted to know what I was doing to celebrate and I replied that I would be going to work, just like I do every day, and then going home to spend time with my lovely wife. I will celebrate when I feel like myself again.

I have had a lot of good feedback from the Inspire.com lung cancer survivor community. I put a description of my diagnosis on the website and asked other patients with a similar diagnosis and treatment to tell me what their experience after chemo and radiation has been. I got four responses, all of which were very positive. Essentially the answer came back...more chemo. The only question really is what drugs to use. It was suggested that I be tested for the EGFR (epidermal growth factor receptor) mutation. If I have the mutation, I might be a good candidate for tyrosine kinase inhibitors such as erlotinib (Tarceva˚). I asked Dr. Scott if the EGFR test has been done. Of course, he had already ordered the test and it came back negative for the mutation.

At the end of my radiation today I met with my radiation oncologist. I asked him how many lung cancer patients he has treated. He estimated that he has treated 10 per month for the past 100 months, since he has been in practice. That would be 1,000 patients or so. I asked about the amount of shrinkage he would expect to get from the treatment I had just finished.

His reply was that there are really two issues — the absolute size of the tumor, and the metastatic activity of the tumor. In terms of size, he said the issue is the volume size of the tumor. Tumor might shrink in size by say 50%, but the VOLUME of the tumor could be significantly more than that — say 75% or even 80%. Even with such shrinkage, the real issue is how active the remaining cells are. This is measured by the SUV value (sugar uptake value), or how much sugar the remaining active cells absorb or take up. The higher the SUV value, the more active the cells, the faster they replicate etc.... At least that is my layman's understanding of it.

My radiologist seems to feel that I have a good chance of being "cured" with my current treatment and he seemed optimistic that my response to the treatment just completed would be good because it was uninterrupted for seven weeks, etc. Anyway, he seemed very positive that the outcome would be favorable. He expects the next step will be consolidation chemo. He did not think that the next "phase" would necessarily be worse than this first round of treatment. I hope he is right.

I kept my blog site knowing that friends, clients, or prospects might eventually read it. I never thought it would happen so quickly.

Apparently someone in my Rotary club did a search on something and the next thing you know, they were reading the blog. Of course, word about my illness spread among my friends like wild fire. The genie is out of the bottle and you can't put her back in.

Yoko is upset that people have found out about this. She does not mind friends knowing, but she does not like the idea of strangers knowing our business. Yoko is sensitive about how the public views our family; she is a very private person and is uncomfortable with having to deal with the people who will naturally ask questions. Yoko expects me to live a long time and she does not want to see any more obstacles put in my way. We have had our share already.

Anyway, it was a bit of a shock to wake up this morning and find out all your friends are clued in to what has been going on for the past few months. I am not sure what the next step should be.

December 15, 2007 — Being Honest

Wednesday morning the proverbial cat was out of the bag and I was receiving phone calls from friends who had found out how sick I am. Of course, they all promised to keep it under wraps, but it is just a matter of time before my cancer diagnosis becomes an open secret, if it is not already.

I am still having trouble eating. I have not felt all that well for the past few days. Aside from the trouble I have eating; I have developed a cough, which I understand may be caused by the radiation irritating my lungs. I feel some heaviness in my chest (like when you have a heavy cold) and worry that I may have caught a cold or that I am developing pleura effusion, which I understand, is common after radiation. I still feel a bit run down and the heaviness in my chest makes me think that there is yet something else going on. I've learned my lesson and will be contacting Dr. Scott on Monday if this does not improve. Actually, I am having a chest x-ray on Monday, so if there is a problem that should help to uncover what it is.

On Thursday I did meet with three clients. None had seen me in months. All three commented that I looked like I had lost weight. (I probably lost 10 pounds.) They asked me if I was OK and, of course, I said I was fine. It made me very uncomfortable to have to lie.

I got a call from Eric Madsen, a long-time friend. He said he considered my daughters and me to be like his own family and he was here to help if we needed anything. It was a nice call to receive. I have gotten a few e-mails from friends as well offering prayers and words of encouragement. I have been busy trying to reply to each.

I am not going to be able to keep this from clients. I am going to have to come clean, but I have not decided yet how to do it.

On Thursday night Yoko and I went to the store to try and get some Christmas shopping done. Suffice it to say I was not feeling great. We spent a very long time looking at cameras and finally selected one to buy. After we made our selection I found out that the price indicated was only about 80% of the real price. To make the camera useful we had to buy additional memory, adding another 20% to the total price. I felt like I had been suckered.

The more I thought about it, the angrier I got. At the checkout, I called the store manager to complain about this sales tactic. I told him selling the camera without the necessary memory was tantamount to selling a car without the engine or wheels. What upsets me is I know this is a purposeful deception aimed at getting people to part with more money than they were planning. It is just a lousy business practice, plain and simple.

My goal has always been to distinguish myself by being an honest and ethical advisor. My good reputation is an asset I vigorously protect. The Rotary four-way test states: Is it the truth? Is it fair to all concerned? Will it build goodwill and better friendships? Will it be beneficial to all? I try to apply the four-way test in all my business dealings. That's why not being up front with people about my health has bothered me so much. Clients and prospects don't necessarily have a right to know about my health, but I feel I am being less than honest by not telling them.

Today we have to finish our Christmas shopping. Yoko, Jessie and I are all going to Fort Myers to see what we can find. Let's hope the merchants there are honest. In my condition, there is no telling what I might do if they aren't!

December 15, 2007 — Hopeful Signs — First Results

I went to see Dr Scott today because I have some swelling around my jaws and a toothache. I think I may have an infection and I don't want it to get worse. He prescribed Amoxicillin 875 mg. to be taken 2 times a day for 10 days. Hopefully this will knock out any infection I may have.

While I was there, Dr. Scott called to get the results of my x-ray. The tumor has shrunk from about 6.8 cm to about 3 cm in diameter (about half the size) which may translate into a larger percentage, in terms of volume.

Again, it is hard to see and measure, but what we know is that the treatment is working as hoped to reduce the tumor size. It is very encouraging news and perhaps the most we can hope for at this stage.

The PET scan, which will give us an idea about the metabolic activity (how active the cancer cells are), will be the real test in January. We had SUV values in the area of 5 to 6, which is highly active. A reduction of SUV values to 2 or so would be a very good outcome. Keep praying. So far so good!

We plan to revisit the question of surgery once more. If Dr. Robinson thought the tumor was now resectable, that would be the very best outcome. I am not too hopeful, but we'll see.

I met with a client who I had not seen for a while. He was somewhat insistent that there must be something wrong with my health and both he and his wife were concerned because I had lost a lot of weight since they had last seen me.

I did not feel comfortable continuing to deny there was a problem, so I decided to confess. In light of all the leaks I felt this would be a good client to "test the waters" and see what his reaction would be. After I told him I had been diagnosed with lung cancer, he said he regretted having pressed me. I explained why I decided to keep this information private and he understood and agreed with my thinking. In fact, he said that I "had nothing to gain by telling clients." Hmmm.... we'll see what happens now.

This particular client will keep the information to himself and is outside the country for more than half the year, so I am not concerned that he will be telling anyone beyond his wife and children.

I found out tonight that the Google search engine picked up anything I had written in my blog. Apparently, the executive director of the free clinic where I volunteer learned about my illness two weeks ago! (He did a search on the clinic name and saw my blog, which referenced the organization.) The rest, as they say, is history.

Who knows how many other searches have turned up my blog. I do know my profile was seen 178 times...two days prior to that it had only been viewed 150 times. (I finally figured out how to eliminate my blog from being searchable as well.) So much for keeping secrets.

December 31, 2007 — New Year Resolutions

OK, so here we are at the start of the New Year. I would like to start this year right and I have been thinking about what my New Year's resolutions should be.

There are a few prerequisites for making a good resolution. First, it should be important. Second it should be within your control. And third, it should be specific and doable. The whole idea of a New Year's resolution is to create a new habit (or break an old bad habit). Usually a resolution will relate to improving your health, finances, or spiritual well being. Last year my resolution was to quit smoking and I finally succeeded! (Too bad I did not have the fortitude to break the habit when I was 20 years old!) The question is, what should be my resolution this year?

I am doing just about everything I can to take care of myself. The one thing Yoko wants me to do (that I am not currently doing) is regular aerobic exercise. (Golf doesn't count.) I am having a hard time committing to aerobic exercise (like running or jogging). I know I should do it, so perhaps using the treadmill for 20 minutes a day should be one of this year's resolutions?

As far as finances, I don't really have any great ideas. We don't have any debt (other than a mortgage, which I plan to keep.) The plan for 2008 is to continue to work, try to increase my income and save 15 — 20% of what I make. I would like to say I will spend less, but with medical bills, college expenses and a wedding coming up, I don't think spending less is in the cards for 2008! I have already committed to donating to our company foundation. They will match my gift and I can commit the full amount to the charity or charities of my choice. I wish I could do more.

In the spiritual realm there are lots of things I should do. Unfortunately I have become a little too cynical about organized religion. I don't have a deeply held belief, but the life example and teachings of Christ inspire me. I would like to try and be more Christ-like in the New Year. Wouldn't it be great if I could inspire good in others by example or bear the trial ahead without complaint? I think if I strive to live like Christ, I will one day be welcomed into heaven. If there is no heaven, I won't know the difference.

One thing I am committed to doing is achieving more with my time. I have always wanted to write a book. I have decided to try and do that in the next year. I have a partially written screenplay on the life of Alexander Hamilton that I want to complete as well. This time next year I hope I can report to you that I have completed both!

The Japanese have a lot of expressions or sayings. One of my favorites is "you eat an elephant one bite at a time." What I need to remember in 2008 is that I can achieve whatever I set out to do if I can make a habit of doing a little bit every day. My New Year's resolution will be to work at all these things one bite at a time.

I am looking forward to a great 2008 and wish for all my family and friends health, happiness and God's blessings throughout the New Year!

Part II — 2008

January 13, 2008 — When You Are Wrong "I'm Sorry" is Always Right

I have been thinking lately about "being right" and "doing right." There are no easy answers to the questions I have. The funny thing is that I am 52 years old and still struggling with issues of right and wrong. Here are a couple of examples of things that have bothered me in the last two days:

Yesterday we are playing golf and the guy I am playing with hits an awful shot into someone's back yard. It is not "out of bounds" because there are no white stakes, so technically, anything is "in play." Anyway, we found the ball and the guy could take a swing. I did not want the guy to play from someone's back yard, so I told him he could take a free drop (no penalty) so that he was not hitting out of the back yard and he said to me, "I don't think the owner is home." In other words, he would play it from where it lays and only take a drop (and technically a penalty) if the owner can see him.

The thought occurred to me that this guy knew it was wrong to be playing the ball from some one's back yard, but he would do it as long as he would not be caught. This guy was formerly the CFO of a very large and well-known public company. I had to wonder what ELSE he did when no one was looking.

Today I was playing golf and hit the ball to the edge of a water hazard. The ball was actually partially in the water but I decided I could play it out, rather than take a drop and a one-stroke penalty. Now technically you cannot touch your club to the ground (ground your club) or touch the water when you are addressing the ball in a hazard. The guy I was playing with is a real stickler for the rules. (To his credit I have to say that he also holds himself to a high standard when it comes to following the rules of golf.)

Anyway, I walked into the hazard and addressed the ball. I was obviously being careful not to touch the water. As I was addressing the ball I inadvertently grazed the bottom of the club to the water (barely enough to even cause a ripple). Before I actually swung my friend said, "That's a two-stroke penalty." He was right, but no one I play with would ever call a two-stroke penalty for what I did, let alone do it before I had hit the ball. (The etiquette (not a rule) in golf is that you call penalties on yourself and you don't talk when someone is addressing the ball.) I made the saving shot and took an 8 (triple bogey) instead of the 6 (bogey).

So here are two situations in two days on the golf course that are kind of similar. What's the point? I guess the point is that the world does not work if we try to run it by rules alone. Rules and laws are broken and sometimes it is RIGHT to break the rules and sometimes it is WRONG. Judgments have to be made about when the rules should apply. The Japanese seem to have figured out that rules and laws are not how members in society should interact. Social norms dominate human interactions in Japan and the society runs very smoothly as a result. In many ways I wish Americans were more like the Japanese.

On my way home from golf some guy in a white Lexus pulled out in front of me and proceeded to do a U-turn in the middle of a the road while I was trying to turn left into the car wash. If I had not stopped, I would have hit him. I raised my two hands and shrugged my shoulders in a gesture of "what the hell are you doing?" Instead of a gesture of "I'm sorry", I was greeted with the middle finger. In the interest of social harmony, a Japanese man or woman would at least have said, "I'm sorry". Here people in the wrong have an "in your face" attitude, that leads to road rage and senseless violence.

Yoko and I are both amazed by how much Americans talk about Jesus and God and then flip the bird to their neighbors. We have to change.

January 16, 2008 — Time for Myself

I am working 12-hour days (on the days that I work) and I still cannot seem to get caught up. The long workdays leaves me little time to do the things I would really like to do. I just wish I had more time for myself.

I have conversations every day with people who make cavalier remarks that just irk me. Someone I was meeting with today (who is roughly my age) said "I want to use my last dollar on the day I die." (With the market down 300 points yesterday, that day may be sooner rather than later!) Anyway, it got me to thinking what a crock this statement actually is...

Look at me! I would STOP working if I knew I am going to die soon. The fact is, I may die this year or next year, or I may live five or ten years. Since I don't know, I have to go on living life the same as I always have and try to maintain and/or grow my bank account. If I get sick, I won't be well enough to spend my last dollar. If I don't get sick, I'll have to keep working.

My lack of enthusiasm for work means I take my sweet time to get into the office. Yesterday morning I was just sitting down to breakfast when the imaging people called to say that the CT/ PET machine has unscheduled maintenance this coming Tuesday. They offered to take me today (if I had not already eaten) or reschedule. Since I had not eaten and had nothing pressing at work, I decided to go in for the CT and PET scan. I got to the place by 10 AM and had an injection of radio isotopes. You have to wait about an hour for these to circulate. Next I had the CT scan, where they inject iodine for contrast and then take a series of high resolution x-rays. After that I had the PET scan.

All I had to do was lie still with my arms above my head while the machine scanned my entire body. It sounds easy. But they were having trouble with the machine. Instead of 25 minutes, I had to lay motionless for nearly an hour. This has never happened to me before and I started to panic. Staying in that machine and not being able to move for that length of time was torture. My arms went to sleep and I literally began to feel something akin to drowning or choking. It was really difficult to complete the test, but, with coaching, I made it through. (This experience does not make me want to go through it again, however.)

I was done with the testing by 12:30 P.M. and took a disc home of the CT pictures, since I did not want to wait to hear the results. There has been obvious dramatic shrinkage of the tumor in my right lung. No wonder I am feeling so good!

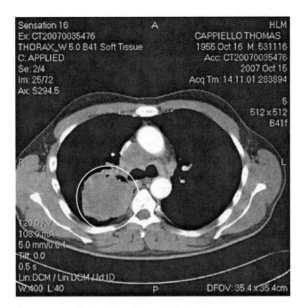

Before treatment the tumor is the size of a baseball.

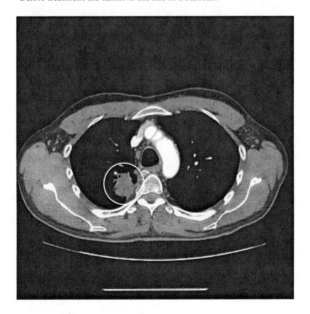

After initial treatment the tumor shrunk 80 percent.

The big question is whether the cancer cell metabolism has slowed. My guess is that it must have or we would not have seen such dramatic shrinkage. I am fully recovered from the first round of chemo. I am golfing in the low 80's again and I have regained weight (now 150 pounds), so I am ready to go on to the next "consolidation" round of chemo.

The shrinkage is so dramatic that it does raise a question in my mind as to whether surgery may now be possible. I will be anxious to ask that question at my next appointment.

The only bad thing about all this good news is that I may have to work for a long time yet. Oh well, I guess that is the price of success? Maybe they will be able to operate and I will get two or three months off work. Let's hope.

January 21, 2008 — To Cut or Not to Cut

I just returned from my appointment with Dr Dave, who is the radiation-oncologist that has been treating me thus far. I brought the CT and PET scans with me to the appointment. Dave's view was pretty much the same as mine; that I had about as good a response to the treatment as one could hope. The question now is what comes next.

What I learned from Dr. Dave is that there appears to still be metabolic activity within the primary tumor, but thus far it does not appear that the cancer has spread. (The radiologist who did the CT and PET, will be providing a report with a more detailed analysis, but that was Dave's best (albeit cursory) read from the pictures.)

Dr. Dave believes that the course of action to give me the best long-term prognosis would be to remove the remaining tumor, if that is possible. While I was there Dave called the thoracic surgeon, Dr Lary Robinson, at Moffitt Cancer Center. I am going to have another appointment with Dr Robinson ASAP and have him look to see if his view (about surgery) has changed. From Dr. Dave's conversation, it sounded as though the option of surgery still remains in considerable doubt. The issue appears to be the location and size of the tumor and now scarring. The fact that we did definitive radiation (7 weeks) vs. a less intensive 5 weeks makes surgery more difficult. If we are going to do surgery at all we have to do it soon; otherwise scar tissue (from radiation) will be the deciding factor.

Dr. Dave's opinion was that I might currently be a borderline surgery case, so it is worth pursuing. We are going to set up an appointment to see Dr. Robinson. If he decides after all to do the surgery, we would do it right away at Moffitt Cancer Center in Tampa. In my case we might have to remove the entire right lung, rather than do a partial re-section. Removing the entire lung, according to Dr. Robinson, is high risk with high mortality from post-operative complications. Moreover, surgery would entail a prolonged (two or three month) period of recovery (assuming you survive the initial trauma!) and would result in significantly reduced breathing capacity.

The other thing Dr. Dave said was that, they could go in to do the surgery and decide, after seeing what's what, that it can't or shouldn't be done! Then I would have to go through all the pain and recovery for nothing!

Frankly, all this does not get me excited to run out and have surgery, especially because I am feeling so well right now! Dr. Dave believes that, whether I have surgery or not, I should proceed with the consolidation chemo. The only problem I have with that recommendation is that I wouldn't want to be in a rundown condition (i.e. anemic or prone to infection) when I go under the knife. I would want to be in excellent shape, which I think would rule out consolidation chemo until we have a final decision on surgery.

Anyway, where we left it is that I will make an appointment to see Dr Robinson at Moffitt ASAP. My appointment with Dr Scott is next week. I would like to see Dr Robinson after I have seen Dr. Scott so I know what questions to ask.

We should have some answers shortly about where we go from here. In the meantime, I am going to relax at home, eat, read, and generally enjoy my current good health! I definitely want to wait on proceeding to next steps until after the Super Bowl!

January 23, 2008 — The Poseidon Adventure

Do you remember the 1972 movie The *Poseidon Adventure* with Shelly Winters, Ernest Borgnine and Gene Hackman? If not, let me remind you of the story line. A passenger cruiser transiting the ocean is suddenly capsized by a gigantic wave. Many of the passengers survive the initial trauma and then try to make their way to the surface in the upside down ship. Of course, most of the passengers tragically die in the process and there is unexpected trouble and disappointment along the way. The route to the surface is debated and different paths are chosen. Only a few ultimately survive, but we learn a lot about the character of each victim along the way.

It seems to me that my cancer experience thus far closely follows the story line of the Poseidon Adventure. Yoko and I had just begun to enjoy our "cruise" toward retirement, looking forward to the next long and uneventful passage in our lives, when suddenly everything is turned upside down by my unexpected diagnosis of lung cancer. The diagnosis was like getting hit by a gigantic wave. After the initial shock and confusion, the panic subsided and we settled down to think more clearly. It is a crisis that tests our faith in God, but we have come to realize we are not in immediate danger of drowning and that we can manage our lives in an upside down ship for quite some time. Just as we began to get our bearings and make our way to the surface, there is another event and more turmoil and we again have to face life and death decisions. Luckily, we have Dr. Scott, playing Gene Hackman's role as Reverend Frank Scott, the compassionate character guiding us to safety!

Why am I telling you all this? Well, I learned today from the Reverend Scott that the PET scan turned up something that is a potential hot spot on my liver. Lung surgery would be off the table if the cancer metastasizes and shows up elsewhere. The "hot spot" the radiologist found may just be a remnant from the radiation (let's hope) but, Dr. Scott, in an abundance of caution, wants to do an MRI to find out for sure. So tomorrow I will have an MRI done. The radiologist will be able to get a better look at what we are dealing with; if in fact it is cancer, the course of treatment (our route to the surface) will have to change.

For me, making it to the surface would be a finding that there is no longer evidence of disease (i.e. the cancer is in remission.) That might happen after surgery or consolidation chemo; a metastasizing disease ("mets") will be a roadblock in getting there. It is part and partial to lung cancer and is to be expected. After all, the ship is upside down ...we have to expect a setback or two. I am confident the MRI will prove the spot to be nothing — but we'll know one way or the other in short order.

I must tell you I feel very comforted to know so many people are praying for me and if asked, would do anything to help. I have had any number of friends (who know about this) stop by the office, come for lunch, invite Yoko and me out to dinner, etc. and offer words of encouragement and support.

Unfortunately, there is a sea of capsized ships out there; many lives are turned upside down. Many people are not as lucky are we are. Millions of other people may one-day get the diagnosis that I have today. How can they be helped?

Lung cancer awareness must be increased and research aimed at early detection has got to be funded. Finding the disease at an early stage will be the key to survival for millions of Americans ((both people with and without a smoking history)) who have not (yet) contracted the disease. There is promising technology out there. Friends and family of lung cancer patients are the ones who will have to carry the flag, since their loved ones with lung cancer have their hands full trying to survive.

January 28, 2008 — Surgical Strike Out

I received word yesterday that the MRI did NOT turn up any more cancer. I was concerned that if I have metastases in the liver, lung surgery would definitely be off the table.

We had a fitful night of sleep last night, so neither Yoko nor I were well rested when we set off for The Moffitt Cancer Center at 6:50 this morning. Unlike our last trip up to Moffitt, we were in and out quickly. We met with Dr. Robinson, who reviewed my most recent CT and PET scans with us, comparing these with the scans done in October. The conclusion is that, despite the tumor shrinkage, surgery is still NOT possible. Dr Robinson explained that the tumor goes from the right lung into the central chest and almost extends into the left lung. He said I was classified as Stage IIIA. However I would be Stage IIIB if the tumor went only a little further and entered my left lung as well.

The radiation and chemo have done a good job shrinking the tumor. In fact, the lung tumor could be removed, but the part of the tumor involving a central chest lymph node can not, making surgery altogether useless. The good news is that the shrinkage in my central chest relieved the superior vena cava, which was being closed off and might have done considerable damage. Dr. Robinson believes that consolidation chemo is the best course of treatment going forward and is currently my best hope for a cure.

Dr. Robinson explained that the removal of the right lung, if it could it be done, has a 30% mortality rate. (That's like jumping out of a plane knowing there is a one in three chance that your parachute won't open!) I asked why the mortality rate was so high and the explanation I received is that the operation requires pinching off the bronchial tubes. In many cases, post-operative complications arise because radiated bronchial tubes do not heal well and a bronchial fistula (leakage) develops.

Actually, I spent a good part of the day yesterday researching and reading about the proposed procedure and the more I read, the more apprehensive I became — ergo my sleeplessness. Besides the 30% chance of dying from the operation and losing a lung, there would also be the possibility of losing my voice entirely, having a heart attack or having other coronary problems. The procedure is also very painful requiring a long (2 — 3 month) recovery period and there is no guarantee that you would enjoy a good quality of life following such a procedure. (Frankly, I am more afraid of pain and becoming disabled than I am of dying!)

Yoko and I will meet with Dr. Scott tomorrow to decide on next steps. Dr. Scott has been thinking about what the treatment should be. There are different schools of thought; some people advocate changing the chemicals used; others would argue for more of the same — emptying both barrels, so to speak, on the cancer.

Emotionally I like the "empty both barrels" approach. The problem is that we have to fight this cancer like a chess game — thinking several moves ahead and not just making the emotionally satisfying decision. We need to consider what our options will be if the cancer pops-up elsewhere down the road. If we use all our ammunition now (Cisplatin and Taxol) there is the possibility that we won't be able to use it later (because of toxicity) or it won't be as effective.

Dr Scott is an excellent doctor and I am an excellent patient. Together we will figure out the best way forward. In the meantime, Yoko and I are planning our June trip to California for Paula's wedding and a September cruise in the Mediterranean. My plan is to be cancer free by summer.

January 29, 2008 — The Verdict on Consolidation

Yoko and I met with Dr. Scott today to discuss what the next steps should be. We are going to continue the chemo using a drug called vinorelbine (Navelbine®) together with Cisplatin. The consolidation treatment is going to go for 16 weeks. We plan to follow the regimen of a study that was published in the New England Journal of Medicine in the June 23, 2005 edition.

We will start the new regimen on Friday, February 15 and continue every Friday until May 30. According to Dr. Scott, the biggest possible side effect from the new drug regimen will be neuropathy (loss of feeling) in the extremities, which happens in about half the cases. The longer the chemo goes on, the more likely it is that I will experience some neuropathy. Other than that, as far as side effects, we would not expect that this course of treatment would be much different than the initial round.

Now how did Dr. Scott arrive at recommending this course of treatment? Well, I think Dr. Scott would be the first to say that we are in uncharted waters. The fact of the matter is no one knows what will work for someone like me. In fact, we can't even say with certainty what caused my tumor to shrink...the radiation, the Cisplatin/Taxol, or the two modalities in combination. In fact, from what I have gathered so far, it appears to me the treatments being used on lung cancer patients today have developed on a hit or miss basis (i.e. constantly trying different things to see what works). So, having said that, one could argue that there is no "right" answer and there is no "wrong" answer regarding the treatment regimen following definitive chemo and radiation.

Here's what we do know. If I do nothing, it is very likely that I will, sooner or later, see a recurrence. How likely is a recurrence? There is perhaps a 70% or 80% chance. If I do have a recurrence, I am not likely to survive it. Another way of saying it is I could do nothing and have a 20 — 30% chance of never seeing any cancer again. In fact my cancer may already be dead and gone and any further treatment might be unnecessary. The sad fact is that there is no way to know that for sure. We have to assume there are still some living cells floating around in my system and that I am in danger of recurrence. The goal, therefore, is to kill these other remnant cells (or keep them from reproducing) wherever they may be lingering using a systemic treatment.

Dr. Scott's thinking in making the recommendation is to treat me as though I had surgery to successfully remove the tumor. If you read the New England Journal article, you will see that the regimen he proposes was tested on a population of early-stage non-small cell lung cancer patients. The drug combination was tested on patients who had surgery to remove the cancer. There were a total of 482 patients in the study. What the study found was that overall survival was prolonged in the chemotherapy group in comparison to the observation group by about 20 months (94 months vs. 73 months). Five-year survival rates for patients with surgery and then the chemo regimen was 69%. The study found that vinorelbine plus Cisplatin has an acceptable level of toxicity and prolonged disease free and overall survival rates.

These statistics are significantly better than what I have been reading about erlotinib (Tarceva˚) and other consolidation drugs, where the "extended survival" was only one or two months — hardly worth the trouble. I think Dr. Scott's suggested course is about as elegant a solution as you are going to find in the circumstances.

Vinorelbine apparently interferes with cancer cell division; Cisplatin works to interferes with the DNA of rapidly dividing cells, including tumor cells, and causes these cells to die. So, I guess if you can kill whatever living cells are still in my system and keep these cells from reproducing, you are going to be better off. At least that is the hope.

February 8 — How to Triumph Over Cancer

I have been having a hard time lately feeling comfortable. I am, frankly, not sure exactly what the problem is and it is hard to describe. First of all, the skin on my upper torso (front and back) is sensitive, as though I had sunburn. It is not really painful, so much as "sensitive" the way your skin becomes sensitive after sunburn. I am pretty sure this is from the chemo.

The other discomfort I am having is tightness in my chest and abdomen (just below the rib cage). The best way to describe it is my abdomen is constantly feeling tight, the way you might tighten you stomach in anticipation of a punch. It feels tight in my chest, like I have something constricting my chest when I breathe. I am thinking that this could be the scarring post radiation and that maybe stretching exercises or some sort of physical therapy would help.

The fact that I am feeling these symptoms now is rather strange, since I finished my radiation treatment two months ago. If I were to have symptoms from radiation, I would have thought the symptoms would show up during treatment.... I have had these symptoms for a while, but they are more noticeable now than they were a few weeks ago.

At Yoko's insistence, I asked Dr. Scott about this and he is stumped. He asked Dr. Dave (my radiation oncologist) as well. I have an appointment to see Dr. Dave next Thursday, but I think I will call and try to see Dr. Scott sooner as this discomfort has become noticeably worse. Yoko thinks it could be that the chemo is beginning to wear off. I did notice that I lost facial hair during chemo. In the past few weeks the facial hair above my lip has started to fill in (darker than before). I looked pretty strange for a while. So maybe Yoko is right. Hopefully, we'll figure it out soon. My new chemo regimen starts this coming Friday February 15.

On Thursday Yoko and I went to a company-sponsored training event in Miami. Thursday evening was a reception and dinner. One of the speakers was Janet Evans, the four time Olympic gold medalist. Janet showed clips of her beating the East German swimmers and setting world records in distance swimming in the 1988 Seoul games. Janet carried the Olympic torch into the stadium during the opening ceremony of the 1996 games in Atlanta. If you recall, she was the one who handed the torch to Muhammed Ali, who lit the Olympic flame that year.

Evans was the event's motivational speaker. She spoke about the difference between being a "winner" and a "champion". She talked about how great athletes develop the right mental attitude when facing adversity. (As she spoke I thought about the mental toughness of Tiger Woods, who is one of the greatest golf champions of all time, and Lance Armstrong, who has beaten testicular cancer and has won seven Tour de France races.) In her career Evans was pitted against the much larger, steroid enhanced East German swimmers. She was an underdog who overcame the odds to become an Olympic champion. It was a good talk and an interesting story. I hope that I can keep a positive mental attitude to overcome the odds facing me.

Friday afternoon, we met Eric and Diane Madsen (lifelong friends who lives in Boca Raton) for dinner at a place called Lola's on Harrison in Hollywood, Florida. Eric has been reading my blog and knew I had just seen an out-of-network ear, nose and throat specialist to get a baseline hearing exam. The bill for looking in my ears and sending me on to an audiologist was a shock. As we sat down to dinner Eric immediately suggested that, "What you SHOULD have done when the ENT said the bill was $360 was say.... eh? What? I can't hear you!"

That is how the entire evening was spent...laughing and joking. Eric gave me just the lift I needed to get me through the next phase of treatments.

February 11, 2008 – Meds to Treat Nerve Pain

I called Dr. Scott today to see if I could book an appointment. Dr. Scott could not see me so we spoke by phone. The long and short of it is that we don't know what may be causing my discomfort, but Dr. Scott believes it could be several things. It could be shingles or it could be the onset of neuropathy or it could be something else. I got the sense that Dr. Scott is inclined to think it may be the start of neuropathy, but he has not ruled anything out.

Shingles (the chicken pox virus) would make sense. It is common for cancer patients to develop shingles because of a rundown immune system. If you have had chicken pox as a kid (and I did) the virus lays dormant in your body. Most people don't get chicken pox a second time. However, anyone who has had chicken pox has the potential to develop shingles, because after recovery from chicken pox, the virus settles in the nerve roots. According to an article on shingles that I found "at risk for shingles are people with leukemia, lymphoma, or Hodgkin's disease, and those whose immune systems have been weakened because they are HIV-positive, or have undergone chemotherapy, radiation, transplant surgery with immunosuppression, or treatment with corticosteroids." The latter category would apply to me.

I put out on the Inspire.com website a description of my symptoms and someone came back to me almost immediately and said it could be shingles. I guess shingles is fairly common among cancer patients. We don't know that this is what I have, but it is possible. From what I have read shingles is no picnic and can become serious, depending on what nerves the virus attacks. Dr. Scott has given me a prescription of Valtrex (an anti-viral), that I will take three times a day for the next seven days. If it is shingles, the Valtrex should give me some relief.

The other possibility is neuropathy. This is perhaps more common and why Dr. Scott seemed more inclined toward this possibility. I have not been able to discern much about neuropathy, other than that it is very common in chemo patients. Neuropathy is characterized by sensations of pain, tingling, burning, numbness, or weakness that usually begin in the hands or feet. It can be caused by certain illnesses, for example, diabetes. It can also be a side effect of treatment with platinum-based chemotherapy drugs. The M.D. Anderson Cancer Center is currently doing clinical trials on how to treat patients with neuropathy, which is an indication of just how common this side effect is. Dr. Scott has prescribed a drug for me called Lyrica, which is an anti-seizure medication often used for patients with fibromyalgia or diabetic nerve pain (DNP). Lyrica is also used for nerve pain after shingles.

Chemotherapy-induced peripheral neuropathy can be either acute or chronic. Acute peripheral neuropathy may begin during or shortly after administration of a platinum-containing drug and usually goes away on its own after several days. Chronic peripheral neuropathy may arise weeks or months after chemotherapy treatment and may be very difficult to treat. In some patients, it may be irreversible. Let's hope that is NOT what I have. I would rather have shingles!

February 14, 2008 — Breast Implants on Valentine's Day

I got a novel Valentine's Day gift today — a breast implant to be inserted tomorrow. Don't get excited, it's not what you think. I am having a "central line" put in my chest so that the nurses have an easier time accessing my veins for chemo and blood work. Getting a central line (a port) is pretty standard procedure for cancer patients facing a long treatment regimen. I think sixteen weeks qualifies.

Actually, my sister Jane (who is a RN) was asking about it. Jane asked if I was getting a central line and was somewhat surprised when I told her that we had not discussed this with Dr. Scott since I was first diagnosed in October. She said that vinorelbine is nasty stuff that should be administered through a port. So, this morning I spoke with Dr. Scott about it and he agreed. He called and we arranged immediately to have it done by my good friend (from Rotary) Dr. John, who is Chief of Staff at Fawcett Memorial Hospital. (By the way, you will not be surprised to know that Dr. Scott has been calling me twice a day (morning and evening) to see if the medication for shingles/neuropathy is working. I am happy to report that it is. I am 80% better than I was on Monday.)

Dr. Scott called Dr. John while I was waiting on the phone. I could only hear what Scott was saying but the conversation made me chuckle and went something like this: "This is Scott calling for Dr. John....Oh, he's in surgery? Can you put me through to him in there? (Long Pause) Hey John, this is Scott. What kind of surgery are you doing this morning....Oh really? (Pause) No... I could never be a surgeon. I'm too short and I'm afraid I might sneeze on the patient... Hey listen, Tom Cappiello, a friend of yours, needs a port. Can you squeeze him in today or tomorrow?"

After Dr. Scott made the arrangements I went to Dr. John's office this morning to do the paperwork; I go under the knife tomorrow morning at 8 AM. This is an outpatient procedure that should take only about 30 minutes. I get something that will put me out.

John tells me I won't feel or remember anything. I told John that my main concern was that the device not interfere with my golf swing, at which point we began to examine my swing to discover the optimum point of insertion! With any luck, this little procedure may actually IMPROVE my game.

I will go to chemo directly from surgery. To be honest, I am glad to be restarting chemo. I like the quiet time it gives me while I get my infusion. So tomorrow, after getting the port, I am headed to Dr. Scott's shop for my first consolidation treatment. The timing of this all worked out very well. Everything gets done on a Friday, giving me one day to recover. With any luck, I can be out on Sunday morning testing out my new swing. If not, I have off on President's Day, which is Monday. Thankfully, I don't expect to get any gifts on President's Day!

February 12, 2008 — How to Deal with Life's Curveballs

My sister Peggy asked me to write about how to deal with life's curveballs. To be honest, I don't feel all that down or worried. It is what it is. What's the use in complaining? I will do what I can (within reason) to treat and deal with the cancer and whatever other illness I have, but it is not going to stop me from living and I am not thinking about it and worrying about it. I am busy living my life every day.

I may not be religious, but I have a fairly strong faith in God. When I die, I know I will be going to a better place. It does not bother me and I am not worried. Writing has been the best therapy for me to deal with my emotions and help me stay positive. Writing gives me time to think out loud and to stand back and consider the situation. I am truly not worried about myself or about what happens to me. I worry most about Yoko and the girls. If I am not here to help and protect them, who is going to do it? It is hard to imagine my family without me in it.

I am relying on having a good mental attitude. I think your mental attitude has a lot to do with how you feel both physically and how you feel about life in general. I decided at the start that I am not going to let cancer run my life or deter me from doing the things I want to do. I am expecting to have lots of trials as this thing progresses. I just have to be mentally tough and work on making myself mentally prepared.

Someone wise once told me that I should only worry about the things I can control. I have taken that to heart and I don't worry about things I cannot change. I try to be prepared. Plan for the worst and hope for the best. I am focused on the things I CAN change or make better. Those are the things I do for my family, friends, community and business.

One technique to keep me positive is focusing on how much worse things COULD be and then thanking my lucky stars that things are not THAT bad. I could have developed lung cancer a long time ago when I was down on my luck! I could have been diagnosed at a later stage when "cure" would not be possible. I could be dealing with this without proper insurance to pay for my treatment. I could be alone in the world with no family support. I could have lousy doctors. I could have had no positive results from my treatments to date. This could have happened at a time when there was no technology or drugs to deal with it. I could have been disabled by the tumor before it was found. I could have had allergic reactions to the drugs that are saving my life. The list goes on and on. Life can be a lot worse…so be thankful for the blessings you have and appreciate your good luck! If I have shingles or neuropathy and this is as bad as it gets, then I am blessed.

We are all going to die one day and our life is only for an instant in infinite time. We have to make the most of the time we have on earth. When you have been diagnosed with a terminal disease, you begin to focus more on what your life is or has been about. Lately I have been thinking about how the things we do have a positive impact on people's lives. Happiness and peace is about fulfillment and satisfaction. I feel very happy because I am fulfilled and satisfied with my life.

Life would not be as much fun if we knew what was coming next. Think of life's little curve balls for what they are — a challenge that keeps us playing and hopefully enjoying the game. We may hit a home run or strike out. Either way, life will have been fun.

Thursday, February 14, 2008 — Setting Priorities

I remember when I went to work in Japan at the age of 23. I was what the Japanese call a "*moretsu shinnyu shaiin*" which roughly translates "over boiling new employee." These are people who start their new job and do whatever it takes to get the job done well. I was frequently in the office early and stayed late into the night. At Penn State I worked very hard to finish my MBA quickly because I had a family and no money. At Arthur Andersen I would often stay up all night to complete projects on time. I worked like a dog to make Partner. I guess when you are young and motivated and starting a career, there is a certain virtue in being "*moretsu*." Then I started my own business, thinking I could parlay what I had into something substantial. In the end I lost everything — except my family, who helped get me through it all. I learned that the only people who REALLY care for you are family and the only thing that REALLY matters is what you do for them and others.

Now that I have developed cancer and face a significantly shorter life expectancy my priorities have changed. Call it the wisdom of age, but a young person should stop and think before putting body and soul into "getting ahead." My views on this have really changed over the past 10 years — since I returned from Japan without a dime to my name. I put so much effort into the work I was doing. Work defined my life. Then I lost it all in a failed business venture. After nearly 20 years of working I had NOTHING to show for all the effort. It occurred to me — do I really want to be defined by what I do to earn a living or is there is something I want out of life that is more important?

I decided the one thing I never want to risk and never want to lose is my family. I decided I want to make the most of my short time on earth and try to get some satisfaction from what I do daily. It just so happens that a friend of mine sent me a 3-minute Internet movie called "The Dash" that says it all. If you have not seen this yet, it is worth watching. Maybe you'll be inspired earlier in life to think seriously about your priorities.

The Dash

In July 2006, a short three-minute movie was launched on the Internet called The Dash. Since then, more than 40 million people from around the world have watched it; and over 20,000 a day continue to watch it as a result of people passing it along.

The movie has been more successful than anyone could have ever imagined. More importantly, however, it has inspired many, many people to reflect on their lives and ask that all-important question, 'Are my priorities where they should be?' I hope you enjoy this movie and share it with those who are close to you.

http://www.dashpoemmovie.com/

Friday, February 15, 2008 — Consolidation Chemo Update

I had the port-placement surgery this morning at Gulf Coast Surgery Center. It is a very nice, modern facility right next to Fawcett Hospital in Port Charlotte. Yoko and I arrived at 8 AM. I filled out paperwork and we were immediately shown a prep room. I changed into a hospital gown and the nurse came in to prep me, which included running an IV of saline and hooking me up to the machine that beeps for your heart rate (84) and automatically takes your blood pressure (111/70) every few minutes. Then, of course, we waited. Every couple of minutes someone would come in and ask a few medical questions, the favorite ones being "did you eat this morning" and "are you allergic to any drugs." Finally, someone came in to say that they were ready to give me a drug that would make me sleep. I remember saying "good" around 9 AM and that's about it. I woke up in the recovery room two hours later.

Yoko took me directly from the surgery center to Dr. Scott's place for chemo. We got there around 11:30 AM. The nurses drew blood and took my weight (160) and I spoke with Dr. Scott briefly. I told him I had the start of a cold and wondered if that would be a problem. He was aware that a bug was going around but he did not seem too concerned and neither am I.

My CBC (complete blood count) is back to mostly normal after taking two months off. My red blood count (RBC) is just slightly below normal. My white blood count (WBC) is right in there on the high end of the range, so I should be OK to fight a cold this week if I need to do that.

As far as today's chemo treatment goes, the drugs they gave me in order were:

- Aloxi 0.25 mg (anti nausea)
- Decadron 20mg (steroid)
- Potassium CL 10 mg
- Magnesium sulfate 500mg
- Mannitol 12.5mg (diuretic agent)
- Cisplatin 60mg (platinum based chemo agent)
- Potassium CL 10 mg
- Magnesium Sulfate 500mg
- Normal Saline 250cc
- Navelbine 40mg (interferes with cell reproduction chemo agent)

I was disappointed not to get any Benadryl. I was looking forward to sitting in the sun and sleeping. This was a 10 bagger and took about five hours to complete. It turned out that one of my clients was being infused. I sat in the chair next to her so there was no hiding the fact that I too am a cancer patient.

Yoko picked me up at the cancer center at about 4 PM and we went directly to the pharmacy to pick up medication for pain, should the incision where I have the port start to bother me. The medication they gave me is oxycodone (the good stuff). I have not taken any, as I am currently pain free.

Yoko made roasted chicken, mashed potatoes, gravy and Jell-O salad for dinner, which was great. I cleaned my plate and feel fine tonight. After dinner, I turned on the TV and fell asleep. I woke up at around 11 PM and am now wide-awake, so I thought I would write.

We have nothing going on this weekend. Tomorrow night we will go to a friend's 50th birthday party. Other than that, the plan is to lie around and see how I am affected (if at all) by the chemo. I am hopeful that this new regimen will work well in fighting off any remaining cancer cells and be safe enough that I can finish it without any of the debilitating side effects. Keep your fingers crossed and say a prayer!

Saturday, February 23, 2008 — One Question I Didn't Ask

I would have been a lousy executive. I remember interviewing for a bank executive-trainee program right after college for The Bank of Virginia (I think). I had made it to the second round of interviews and I remember I had to travel to Virginia from Pennsylvania for this interview. Let me tell you the ending so this doesn't get too long winded. I didn't get the job and I know why I didn't.

We were asked to do role-playing so that the people judging me could tell something about my decision-making skills — that is, my ability to collect relevant information and based on that, make the right decisions. The scenario they gave me had to do with my being a store manager, whose job was to enforce the merchandise return policy. Some lady wanted to return an item (a pair of shoes) that was not within the terms of the return policy and had insisted on speaking to me. Long story short, I interviewed the lady and gathered all of the information. She had made the purchase 60 days ago and our return policy was 30 days. The shoes she wanted to return had obviously been used. No, she did not have a receipt, but yes, it WAS our store brand. After carefully weighing all these and similar pertinent facts, I basically decided to tell the lady she was NUTS. Not only would I not accept this as a return item and refund her money, I would not even give her store credit for a portion of the cost. I was tough. I made an executive decision to turn her down flat. This executive decision making thing was pretty easy!

In my exit interview (where I was NOT asked back) I found out where I had gone wrong. The lady was the daughter of the owner of the store. She was our biggest customer. She had purchased about $10,000 a month in shoes from my department. Hmmm. I never asked about THAT. Yes, in retrospect, I suppose it might have been important to know WHO this lady was…

What does all this have to do with cancer you ask? I guess the bottom line is that I haven't learned much in the intervening 30 years.

My sister Jane is an RN. Since being diagnosed with cancer, I thought she would be a good resource and sure enough she is. Jane seems to know all the latest drugs, etc. In fact, when she heard I was having vinorelbine (Navelbine®), she was the one that suggested a port would be the way to go.

Anyway, tonight Jane and David came down from Philadelphia. We picked them up at the Fort Myers airport around 6:15 P.M. and went to Sanibel for dinner. I was telling Jane at dinner about today's chemo treatment. I told Tammy, the nurse who was giving me my drugs today, that my sister the RN suggested a port. Tammy asked me "what kind of a nurse is your sister?" And I said, "she is an IV nurse; she gives IVs to people in their homes".

Apparently that was the wrong answer. That might have been partly right 10 years ago. Since then Jane's specialty is ONCOLOGY! She is an oncology nurse working at Lehigh Valley Hospital, one of the largest oncology centers in PA! Here is another case of not getting all the facts. I guess her knowing all these cancer drugs should have been a hint! If I could just stop talking long enough to ask one more question — I might have known that! Oh well, Jane thought it was funny, but I thought it was embarrassing!

The restaurant where we ate was La Dolce Vita (an Italian place where Yoko and I went about a month ago). The food was excellent. They have live entertainment, so it was a little noisy. We had a nice time visiting on the way there and on the way home. Tomorrow we head out on a friend's boat, which they have kindly offered. The plan is to go to Boca Grande and eat at a Jimmy Buffet kind of restaurant only accessible by boat…have lunch… hang out on the beach until sunset and then make our way home. The weather should be sunny and warm. It will be a nice break for Jane and David, who had to dust snow off their car before leaving home.

March 7, 2008 — Life in the Fast Lane

These days I feel like I am living in the fast lane and time is just flying by! To add to this feeling, I had steroids today and I am so hyped up I feel like I could run a marathon!

I have not posted to my blog in a week because I have been so busy. What am I doing? Well, we lost our executive director at the free clinic and as Treasurer some of the burden has fallen to me to lend management help. Now that we have a clinic and multiple locations where we are dispensing drugs, the operations have suddenly become more complex and will require some oversight. The first challenge was building and opening the clinic; the ongoing challenge will be funding operations on a continuing basis. On a very low level we need $350k a year to keep the doors open; to operate more meaningfully we are looking at more than twice that amount. In addition to the time at the clinic, I am working to help obtain the funding. I enjoy my clinic role and doing something that has a meaningful impact on people's lives.

I applied to attend the National Lung Cancer Partnership's Advocate Summit in Texas in May. I've decided that I want to advocate for lung cancer research and early detection. We could save or extend millions of lives if we could find a way to catch lung cancer when it is Stage I or II. Your chances of long-term survival are greatly diminished (5% chance to live five years) when you are diagnosed Stage III or IV. Had there been screening available for someone like me, we might have caught my cancer before it developed to Stage III. I feel confident I am going to be in the one-in-twenty "survivor" ranks instead of the "victim" ranks. And because I think I will be a survivor, I feel an obligation to push for research and early detection. If I don't do it, who is going to?

As far as my health goes, my white blood count (WBC) is down to 2.5. We began this round of treatment at 8.8 and normal range is 4.2 — 10. Last week the count was 2.9 and the week before that it was 6.1. It has really dropped more quickly than during the last round of chemo, which was more gradual. I asked Dr. Scott about this and his response was that the bone marrow exhibits more damage as treatment continues. The first round of 8 treatments did not result in this kind of dramatic downturn...but the current treatment has shown the WBC count to fall like a rock. An impaired bone marrow is the answer.

If the WBC gets too low, we won't be able to continue the current treatment until I recover. Staying "on schedule" is important to getting good results. so...Dr Scott is going to give me filgrastim (Neupogen®) shots starting tomorrow at 8 A.M. This is supposed to cause the bone marrow to increase production of white blood cells. He is also concerned that my cold has not resolved so he wrote a prescription for an antibiotic, which I am to take for three days. If I did not have the cold I would feel 100 percent. Even with the cold, I feel 95 percent. I am not tired or suffering any of the usual chemotherapy side effects. My red blood cells are at 4.02, which is low, but just below the normal range of 4.5 — 6.4.

I am scheduled for three shots of Neupogen: tomorrow (Saturday) and then Monday and Tuesday before work. Some people who have had the shots say they made them sick or result in bone pain, so I am a bit apprehensive. Hopefully this new drug, like all the others, will roll off my back and not impact my daily living. I have too much going on to be sick!

March 15, 2008 — A Simple Thank You

One of my favorite lines and monologues in a movie comes from the 1992 movie *A Few Good Men*. Jack Nicholson plays a dedicated Marine colonel stationed in Guantanamo, Cuba who is dragged into court by a JAG defense lawyer played by Tom Cruise."... I want the truth!" Cruise screams as he questions Nicholson on the stand. "You can't handle the truth!" snaps Nicholson, who then goes into a long monologue about "standing on that wall" and defending the country and taking advantage of the freedom he provides. Nicholson ends his diatribe with "A simple 'thank you' will do."

I was at Florida Cancer Specialists this morning at 9 A.M. on the nose. They took my blood and then they guided me into the office to see Dr. Scott. We discussed various things, but the first thing he did was thank me for the letter I sent to him and his staff. They really do a great job and I thought he and they should know it. So I sent a letter of thanks (below).

The Japanese are very diligent about saying "Thank You" and "I'm Sorry". When Americans go to Japan, they rave about Japanese "politeness". They should rave about what is "common courtesy." We need to get that back in this country. There was a time when being polite was important.

Anyway, here is the letter I sent to Dr. Scott and the staff at Florida Cancer Specialists. These people are dedicated and work really hard and do a very good job. I believe they are saving my life. The least I could do is say thank you!

> Dear Dr. Scott and Staff:
>
> Unfortunately for me, as you know, I was diagnosed with Stage IIIA locally advanced adenocarcinoma in October of 2007 and referred to you by my primary physician.
>
> I just want you and all the staff and nurses and management to know how fortunate I feel I am to have you as my medical oncologist, your office staff doing my scheduling and billing, and the oncology nurses (I can name them all) treating me. Not only are you all highly professional and thoughtful about my care and treatment, you demonstrate every day that you truly care about the person being treated. I experience and observe it every time I visit your office — from the moment I walk through your doors to the moment I leave. I would love to be able to someday emulate your professionalism and efficiency in my own practice.
>
> Having spent hours upon hours in your facility, I have had a great opportunity to watch how people are treated when they are greeted, drained, examined, re-poured, and sent on their way with appointments for next time. It is a thing of beauty to watch "the client experience" and the "tailoring" of treatment at your facility. I think many businesses, including my own, could learn from what you seem to do so naturally and so well. Your quality control is impeccable. I am not sure if it is the systems,

the training, the people you hire, the management, or something else. I suspect it is a combination of all the above. Most importantly, your organization exudes a culture of caring. I do see it as very special and something for which you should all take great pride. This is coming from someone who spent a career in Japan, in a society that is acclaimed for being polite and efficient. Let me assure you that the Japanese and their QC methods have nothing on your operation.

It is 5 A.M. and thanks to the steroids you gave me this morning I have not had a wink of sleep. While I was lying awake I was thinking that I would like to do something for you and your staff. The only thing I could think to do is to thank you sincerely and with all my heart. You all do a wonderful job and you should know it.

Yours Very Sincerely,

Tom Cappiello

March 28, 2008 — Finding the "Groove"

I became a teenager during the '60's and one favorite expression of the time was "groovy." Simon and Garfunkel picked up on the fashionable word of the day and put it in a song. I remember how much my mother liked their song and really perked up when singing "Feeling Groovy!" I am not sure I ever really understood what feeling "groovy" was supposed to mean — and I am not sure there is an agreed definition, but I suppose we could assign the meaning to be "feeling good as a result of being in the groove."

After a diagnosis of cancer, your life feels like it is upside down. Your expectations of tomorrow are suddenly changed. You have a new set of worries and concerns. The biggest concern is about "what happens next." No doctor wants to tell you how the disease might progress or what is likely to happen because they don't know. In short, getting a diagnosis of a terminal disease like lung cancer takes you out of your day to day "groove." All of a sudden your daily life is upset. Nothing seems right and nothing you do feels right. All you REALLY want is to get back in the groove of your daily life. Referring to golf, my friend Len said it best. It is like an Olympic bobsled speeding down the track...and all of a sudden when you hit a bump or curve that takes you out — you either recover or you go flying off the track. The goal in golf, bobsledding and dealing with cancer is maintaining your composure and getting back into the groove that will guide you safely to a happy ending.

Here is how I have come to think about my "chances" of beating cancer to get back in the groove. To say you are going to beat lung cancer is like saying you expect tails on the next flip of the coin, even though you have flipped the coin 100 times and it has come up tails only 15 times! In fact, in this example, every flip has a 50 / 50 chance on EACH flip of the coin. There is NO predicting the NEXT flip based on the last 100 flips! (In the parlance of Wall Street — past performance is not indicative of future results!) On the other hand....If you flipped a coin 10,000 times, I would NOT bet that you would get all heads or all tails...I would expect the likely outcome is that I would get 5,000 tails and 5,000 heads or close to those numbers unless the coin was somehow being affected by outside influences (weight, wind, the flipping technique, etc.)

Each cancer case is a flip of the coin. We don't KNOW what the outcome will be, even though we know we have a 50% chance of heads and a 50% chance of tails. (In my case, I have statistically a 15% chance for cure and an 85% chance for no cure.) The outside influences (youth, good performance status, good reaction to therapy, no mets, good doctor, etc.) increase my chances for a cure....let's say to 50%. Now, if I can get in a "positive mental groove" the outcome will be in my favor. This is like trying to make a putt in golf. I can make long putts when I am in the groove and have confidence of making long putts. The same thing applies here. I am glad to report that I am feeling "groovy."

What is the plan for next week? Monday and Tuesday I have to get my shots. Tuesday I have to see the ENT about my hoarseness, which seems to be about the same or a little worse. Otherwise, you could hardly know I am sick at all. The neuropathy seems about the same. I feel numbness in my feet and a little in my fingers. Next Friday will be my eighth chemo in consolidation and will mark the half way point. Hopefully, I can remain healthy and "in a groove" through April as I have a lot to do!

April 6, 2009 — Catching Up

I have actually been writing quite a bit, I just have not posted everything I have written. I have been in a bit of a funk this past week, for no reason that I can easily discern.

It started with my feeling sick over the weekend. After chemo last Friday I was nauseous. I did not work the gates at the Southwest Florida International Air Show, as I normally do, because I did not want to be exposed to thousands of people while my WBC count is low. On Saturday I had the first of three Neupogen shots. Saturday afternoon I played golf. I was feeling nauseous during golf and finally lost it in the bushes around the 7th hole. I blame it on the chemo, but truthfully it might have been the golf. (I shot over 100 for the round that day.) I was not feeling much better on Sunday and my golf improved only slightly.

On Monday I had a Neupogen shot in the morning. In the afternoon Yoko and I went to sign our estate documents. There is a lot of work I need to do to get our affairs in order. The primary culprit is the fact that Yoko is not a US citizen, which complicates things. She is not entitled to the "unlimited marital deduction" that married US citizens are entitled to receive. As a result, any amount exceeding $2 million today that I leave to her as part of my estate (which includes life insurance proceeds) is subject to the estate tax. I am entitled to gift Yoko up to $125,000 per year, so our plan is to gift the things in my name or in joint name to her. In the meantime, we will try and get her citizenship.

All the discussion of death and taxes did not lift my spirits. On Tuesday I got my third shot of Neupogen for the week. At lunchtime on Tuesday I attended the Charlotte Estate and Tax Planning Council, where I listened to more discussion of death and taxes. After the luncheon, which was also held at Kingsway Country Club, I was still not feeling great, so I decided to go home and go to bed. I did not leave bed until late Wednesday morning. Mostly I just slept. (Tuesday night I did finally finish "Team of Rivals," the book on Lincoln that I started when I began chemo last October.)

I decided to take myself off Lyrica (nerve pain medication), with Dr. Scott's permission. If I have nerve pain that comes back, I can always go back on medication, but I am not in the habit of taking drugs unnecessarily and this particular drug affects the brain. I am down now to taking just one pill a day for acid reflux. I have been off Lyrica since Tuesday and feel no worse for it. In fact, I am wondering if the Lyrica could be some of the reason I was feeling depressed.

Now let me tell you the good news. In my meeting with Dr. Scott today, he told me that my CEA (carcinoembryonic antigen, which is a marker in the blood commonly associated with lung cancer — like the PSA is associated with prostate cancer) was back to the normal range. When the cancer was discovered in October, my CEA level was 77 (normal is the 4 — 6 range). In December the CEA was 12 and it is currently 5. That is a good indication that treatments are working. This week I will have three more Neupogen shots and on Wednesday I will have both a CT and PET scan to see what progress we are making. I am not looking forward to the PET scan because of my bad reaction last time. Hopefully, we will find that the cancer is under control.

Friday, April 17, 2008 — Latest Scan Results

I went to get a new PET and CT scan on Wednesday. The purpose of these tests is to monitor the cancer and see if the treatments are working to kill the existing tumor and keep it from spreading. As I write this I am sitting in the sunlight of the solarium getting my 18th chemo infusion (six more to go). I have not heard anything yet about the results of my PET and CT scans. Hopefully, there will be no surprises.

The last time I had a PET scan it took more than an hour. Normally, the scans take 25 minutes, but apparently they had a software upgrade that was causing the machine to crash while I was in it. I became extremely anxious while waiting in the machine. The feeling was the feeling you might have if you were drowning. I almost did not complete the test last time, so I was nervous about doing the test again. This time I brought my i-pod with me and that helped to get my mind off the feeling I was in a coffin.

STOP.....FLASH!

I sent an e-mail to Dr. Scott while I was sitting here getting chemo to let him know I was awaiting the test results. He just came by to personally deliver the good news! The tumor has shrunk to 2.4 X 2.1 cm in size; the SUV (sugar uptake value — a measure of the metabolic activity) is in the normal range of 3.1 and there is no evidence of disease elsewhere! The treatments are continuing to shrink the tumor and, most importantly, reduce the metabolic activity. That is very good news indeed! In fact, it doesn't get any better.

One of the peculiar things that have happened to me is that I am frequently getting leg cramps at night. I will be sleeping and all of a sudden my right calf will cramp, as though I had just run a marathon. Apparently, the chemo can affect the level of potassium in your blood and low potassium can result in muscle cramps. Now here is the weird part. This morning I fell out of bed and hit my face on some glass candle holders that are at my bedside. I cut my nose and lip and bruised my cheek. I THINK I was DREAMING that I had a muscle cramp and jumped out of bed to try and walk it off. But I don't remember anything until waking up on the floor. Yoko observed me jumping out of bed....standing for a second and them collapsing on the floor. (I scared her to death.) So now, in addition to having cramps I will have to determine if the cramps are real or imagined!

May 4, 2008 — Entering the Next Phase

Last Saturday Jessie came home from college and moved back into our house. It is so nice having her home again! I can't believe she is already finished her first year of college! This whole cancer thing started right after Jessie got up to Florida State last fall. The initial shock was such that I was not sure I would even be around for her first year of school or Paula's wedding next month. Luckily, I have responded very well to treatment and I am optimistic that I have more than one or two years ahead of me. Let's hope!

I now have to have Neupogen shots three times a week to build up my white blood cell count so that I can continue treatments on schedule. The shots themselves don't bother me much. They make my bones ache a little and I don't feel quite myself after getting them. This past Friday the nurse said I may need to get Procrit next as my RBC (red blood cell) count is getting low. I have sent a note to Dr. Scott about this as I don't want to show up for treatment next Friday and be told my RBC is too low to get the scheduled infusion. I understand that the Procrit shots can be debilitating for a day or two.

I only have four treatments left — two long ones (Cisplatin and Navelbine, which take five to six hours) and two short ones (Navelbine only, which takes about two hours) and I will be done. My last infusion is on May 30, the day after Project Graduation, a Rotary event I am chairing. The following week we leave for California for Paula's wedding. I don't want the treatments to go off schedule at this point because it would bump into Paula's wedding. I could get treatment in California the day before the wedding, but who wants that! Anyway, we're going to try to stay on schedule so that I am feeling healthy June 7, when I give the bride away!

Yesterday Jessie, Yoko and I went down to Fort Myers. Jessie and I played golf at The Verandah Country Club while Yoko went shopping for stuff we need, including gift cards for Project Graduation! When we got back from golf, Jessie went out with her friends to take pictures of friends going to the high-school prom; Yoko and I went to a charity event — this one to raise funds for housing for homeless kids. There must have been 500 people at the event, called "An Evening in Oz" orchestrated by the Leadership Charlotte Class of 2007 — 2008.

It seemed like we knew at least half the people there — friends from Rotary, the Charlotte Chamber of Commerce, St. Vincent de Paul, people from work, golfing friends, clients, etc. We had a good time. Afterward we went to "Bin 82" which is a new hangout in Punta Gorda being run by one of Paula's friends from high school. At "The Bin" we ran into more friends, including the wife of a friend who has a 53 year old sister with lung cancer. I spoke with her for a while about her sister. She is not doing as well as I am and has had a hard time with the treatments. Another friend's father I spoke with that night has lung cancer. It is everywhere.

I must say, it is satisfying to go to these affairs and see so many people and to know we have so many friends who care about us. I know many of these people will be a huge help to Yoko down the road.

I feel I am at a crossroads entering a new phase of my life and my fight with cancer. I finish chemo on May 30th with no more treatments planned; the following week Paula gets married. In July Yoko and I take a road trip up to Virginia to see Jane and David's lake house and then onto Washington D.C. to begin our lobbying effort to fund lung cancer research and early detection. In the fall we are planning a trip to Italy. There is no time to waste...

May 23, 2008 — Leading by Example

I am more emotional tonight than I am normally. Maybe it's the drugs. A lot of things have happened in the past two weeks. I have not sorted them all out and there is no particular order...so let me just tell you about events and see if you can make the connections.

I was watching the movie *Braveheart* with Mel Gibson tonight. I must have seen it 20 times or more already. In a nutshell, it is about a man named William Wallace, who believes life is not worth living without freedom from tyranny. He inspires his fellow Scots to liberate Scotland from a ruthless English tyrant. In one scene, he speaks to the assembled Scottish warriors, who, are outnumbered by the opposing English forces. The Scots are about to leave the battlefield and admit defeat, before the fight has even taken place. Wallace rallies them by saying, in so many words, that he would rather fight and lose, than not to fight and die years later in his bed having lived a life without freedom. It is an inspiring scene. What inspires I think is Wallace's willingness to lead by example.

I went to a client's home today to witness the execution of his last will and testament. My client is bed ridden, dying from cancer. He fought hard, but God wants him too badly. He was diagnosed in September, only a month before me and elected to have surgery to remove most of his esophagus. He was a New York City fireman who worked the pile on September 11th. He is another Osama Bin Laden victim that you won't read about or hear about. When I saw my friend today, he looked like one of the victims of the Nazi death camps. Bruce and I are the same age. He will be leaving his wife, a grown daughter and son behind. I promised Bruce that I would look after his family finances and I plan to be here to keep that pledge.

I have been reading Andrew Jackson's biography and how he saved New Orleans and the Louisiana Territory from Creek Indians at Horseshoe Bend on the Cumberland River in the early 1800's and later from the British in the War of 1812. At Horseshoe Bend his Tennessee militia were lacking supplies, cold, starving and near mutiny at one point and ready to give up and go home. Jackson was able to rally them. He inspired them with his nationalistic appeals and executed one man (who had not been formally relieved from his post) to make an example of his resolve to maintain discipline. It struck me how easily leaders are willing to take someone's life to make a point. We don't give much thought or notice to the victims of such point-making.

I was talking with a friend of mine, whose sister-in-law has given up on fighting her lung cancer. She is not doing well and she has adopted something of a defeatist attitude. How do you inspire someone to fight a terminal disease? How can you motivate them?

I was invited today to write a column in the "Feeling Fit" section of the Charlotte Sun called "Living with Cancer." I am going to speak with the editor next week and see how much space there will be and how frequently she wants a submission. I plan to use this blog for core material. This is a great opportunity for me to increase lung cancer awareness and hopefully inspire people to live a full life. I am hoping to set an example of how you overcome the odds and beat back the enemy. Surrender is not in my vocabulary.

Speaking of putting up a good fight, I decided to go ahead and enroll in a Phase III Clinical Trial for a drug called Stimuvax. If I participate in the trial, there is a one in three chance I will get a placebo and not the actual drug. On the other hand, that is better than not participating and there is nothing else out there currently that would fit my profile as well.

About this time next week, I hope to be on the road to recovery from all the drugs they have pumped into me these past seven months and in shape both mentally and physically to really enjoy my daughter's wedding day

August 2008 — Brain Radiation and Entering a Drug Trial

On our return from our lobbying effort in Washington D.C. last July, Yoko and I decided to forge ahead with our life together and try to do things we might not have the chance to do later on. We began making travel plans to Europe, something we might never get to do if my health deteriorates. We planned the trip of a lifetime — three weeks in Italy for early October, 2008.

If I have a recurrence of cancer, it is more likely to show up as metastasis to the brain or bones. In the first phase of my treatment, we were dealing directly with the lung tumor to shrink it and kill any metabolic activity. That seemed to have worked. In the second phase of my treatment we were trying to deal with the cancer systemically — that is, to kill any cancer cells that could be floating around in my body and showing up as metastatic cancer, say to the liver or kidney. The problem, however, is that chemo does not work so well in the brain. Lung cancer patients will frequently develop secondary brain tumors, despite having been treated with chemo. This tendency for chemo not to help with brain tumors is said to be the result of "the blood-brain barrier". Given the size of my tumor at diagnosis, I felt I was at risk to develop brain tumors. I am more afraid of being disabled by brain tumors than of dying.

I spoke with Dr Scott as well as my radiology oncologist about the idea of doing whole brain radiation as a preventative. I also did research on the Internet and called on online support groups to give me advice. The bottom line was that there is no research to suggest that it helps and there is no research to suggest that it does much long term harm. Nevertheless there are dangers to radiating the brain, such as seizure from brain swelling due to the radiation, potential memory loss, etc. The other risk is that, if down the road I did develop mets to the brain, whole brain radiation as a treatment would be off the table as the brain (or any organ for that matter) can only take so much radiation.

After a lot of handwringing I decided to go ahead with brain radiation. We determined to do 15 treatments — roughly half the radiation I had in the lung. Given the lack of hard evidence either way, my thinking about this was simple. If I don't do it and I develop brain mets, I will have wished I had. If I develop brain mets anyway, what did I lose? I decided that I would rather go down fighting than regret not having done everything possible.

I also decided to enter into a clinical trial — a double blind study — for a drug called Stimuvax. This is one of the only drug trials for lung cancer currently underway. If I got into the trial, I had a two-thirds chance of getting the actual drug, rather than a placebo. The problem was that I had to "qualify" for the trial, which required that I be a Stage III non-small cell lung cancer patient who is "stable" and begin the trial within 12 weeks of completing chemo. In order to enter the drug trial within 12 weeks of finishing chemo, I had to start the receiving the drug by the end of August. That meant I had to squeeze two weeks of brain radiation in the last two weeks of July. Our trip to Italy was planned for October.

Part III — 2009

Lack of Research Funding for Lung Cancer

Isn't it interesting that I had treatments for nearly one year to deal with the large tumor in my right lung, but there was only "evidence based treatment" for the initial eight weeks of treatments I received? After completing chemo-radiation in December of 2007 — two months after my tumor was discovered — there was nothing more evidence-based medicine could do for me. Dr. Scott liked to say "we are in uncharted waters" when it came to doing anything further. "Are you kidding me? That's it? "I was astounded that there was not more I could do.

No one knows what modality of treatment has worked for me — the adjuvant chemo and radiation first line treatment I initially received, the 16 weeks of consolidation chemo of Cisplatin and Navelbine, the whole brain radiation, or the clinical trial drug I am now taking. No one can predict if I will stay healthy or relapse. When it comes right down to it, there is not much we know about why I have done so well. Maybe it is something in my genes? (If that is the case, I should bottle it and sell it!)

I find it amazing that after decades of "the war on cancer" we are virtually no further along in treating the number one cancer killer — lung cancer — than we were in 1971. Can you imagine if computer technology had not progressed since 1971? There would be no such thing as a personal computer or wireless phones or texting or the Internet.

Why are we able to make great strides when it comes to the futuristic technology we employ in our daily lives today (GPS navigation, digital voice recognition, satellite TV, mobile phones, etc) but can't seem to get to first base when it comes to the biology of cancer? Could it be that in our quest for safety and the regulatory environment has created gigantic speed bumps making the cost of developing new technology prohibitive?

Imagine how slow cell phone technology would have developed if the FDA required that we test the phones to see if prolonged use will result in brain tumors. I dare say we would not have seen cell technology develop at the spectacular speed it did. We would all be walking around with eight pound monster phones. We would not have the lung cancer epidemic we have today if the FDA had regulated tobacco companies. How much testing did we do before cigarettes were allowed on the market?

In April of this year I attended a conference put on by the National Lung Cancer Partnership called the National Lung Cancer Advocate Summit in Dallas Texas. The conference was intended for people like me who want to do something about the lack of awareness and funding for lung cancer. Researchers from the University of Texas provided us with a one day course to explain what is known about the biology of cancer and what is yet to be learned. Suffice it to say that, while we know a lot about the complexities of the various forms of cancer, there is much more that we don't know. Research dollars need to be devoted specifically to lung cancer.

The Healthcare Reform Debate — My Two Cents

The debate about healthcare reform is raging on and it has a lot of people concerned about the future direction of the country. I feel I am (or should be) on the front lines of the debate. First of all, I am a lung cancer patient receiving excellent care from our privately run health system. I wouldn't change that for the world. On the other hand if I lost my job I would be one of the people who would be uninsurable. Secondly, I am Chairman of the Board of the Virginia B. Andes Volunteer Health Clinic, a not-for-profit clinic and pharmacy here in Charlotte County, which is taking care of the needs of thousands of people in our community who have no healthcare coverage, including patients with cancer. I have a pretty good idea about who the uninsured are. Third, I've lived in a country that has universal healthcare (Japan), so I know what is possible. And lastly, being a stockbroker, I understand how markets work. I feel I understand the issues in the debate — both pro and con. Would you like to know what I think?

Having the central government command a crucial part of our economy can be likened to my experience in China in the mid-1980s. At the time I was working with the accounting firm Arthur Andersen. We were engaged to help one of the world's largest producers of duck decide whether it was the right time to invest in China. The Chinese did not produce enough duck and wanted my client's technology so they could produce more. After a 10 day trip to understand the environment we did not go forward with the project because the Chinese had a political need to control poultry prices and would not allow us to charge what it cost to produce ducks and receive a premium for the risk we would be taking. The government ran the show in China and could not politically do what was needed to increase pricing to attract producers and create a clearing market. The result was price controls and a continuing shortage of duck. It's the same reason there were bread lines in Russia.

Today we have the equivalent of breadlines in the healthcare industry. We have a dwindling supply of primary care physicians because they are not sufficiently reimbursed from the government run insurance provider, Medicare (i.e. price controls). The supply of healthcare providers is shrinking because of cost controls imposed by government and private insurers. Once everyone has "universal healthcare insurance" and cost becomes irrelevant there will be lines for every kind of healthcare service. That's just the nature of markets. What we need to make our healthcare system work is a clearing market — equilibrium between supply and demand.

Frankly I am not sure insurance is the answer. When someone else (an insurer) is paying virtually the entire cost, what incentive is there to keep costs down? We'll spend whatever it takes to keep Mom and Dad alive, even if it is for a few more weeks. That doesn't make much sense really.

I think the answer is staring us straight in the face but no one has proposed it. We should have public facilities, just like we have public schools. We have made education a human right and mandated that every community have public schools. Why couldn't we do the same thing for healthcare? Couldn't we create public health clinics and dental clinics, out-patient surgery centers, imaging centers and hospitals where you can be treated for free? There is no need for an insurance intermediary. Undoubtedly, since it is free, there would be lines. And we would need an army of doctors to do their residency and hone their skills at these public facilities. We could have a system where, after a certain period of low-paying public service, medical student's school loans are paid by taxpayers and forgiven. Doctors could then enter into private practice debt free. Any healthcare worker working at a public facility would be entitled to sovereign immunity and indemnified by the state. We already do this at the free clinic.

If you don't like the quality of services a public healthcare facility provides (and I am not saying it would be good), nothing would stop you from purchasing health insurance and going to private facilities and paying a premium for superior service.

How would all this be paid for? What about using the $900 billion President Obama is saying we can save from the waste in the current system to build healthcare facilities all over the country? (This would be a stimulus on par with the building of the national interstate road system and a gigantic stimulus to the economy.) We should be able to divert Medicare insurance proceeds to building a public healthcare system. Medicare recipients would have to use public facilities. We're still going to end up with a shortage of healthcare workers, but I am sure we could create incentives to create the added workforce we will need.

Fighting the Stigma of Lung Cancer

Something happened the other day that I am ashamed to tell you. I snapped. Here's what happened. I went over to the Punta Gorda office of State Representative Paige Kreegle to pick up the proclamation made by Governor Crist declaring November "Lung Cancer Awareness Month" in the state of Florida. I was talking with his administrative aide, who had kindly done the work necessary to get the Governor to make the proclamation and I found myself yelling at him for a passing comment he innocently made as I was leaving the office. The comment was something to the effect of "Yeah, Paige can really get behind this (Free to Breathe 5K lung cancer awareness) event. He hates smoking." It was the last three words that set me off. "This is not about smoking," I said, "it's about LUNG CANCER!"

I tried to straighten out the young man, by explaining something to him. I should have been calmer, but it raised the hair on the back of my head and I let go.

Here are some facts that nobody wants to say out loud. Yes, we all want to see people quit smoking. Smoking is not good for you and is ONE OF the direct causes of lung cancer, as well as other cancers, other lung disease and heart disease. (Radon is also KNOWN to be a direct cause of lung cancer.) We need to make sure that young people never start smoking and avoid the addiction. Once you start, believe me, it is a very difficult drug habit to break.

But the fact is that, even had I quit 10 or 20 years ago, I would STILL have had an elevated risk for developing lung cancer. Quitting does NOT eliminate the risk. That fact, of course, is not well advertised because, if long time smokers believed that they are going to contract lung cancer anyway, why quit? I understand the logic. The problem is that, because smoking is blamed for causing lung cancer, we are not investing in research for early detection and treatment. Lung cancer is seen as a self-inflicted disease, not really worthy of public research funding. The sad fact is that lung cancer is the No. 1 cancer killer, with one of the lowest survival rates. Yet it gets the least amount of the available cancer research funding. Explain that to me.

This year there will be more than 200,000 new cases of lung cancer diagnosed. Something like 10% — 15% of the new cases will be people who NEVER smoked. That is 20,000 to 30,000 cases a year. More than 100,000 of the new cases will be former smokers (people who quit prior to their diagnosis). So if you take these two groups together, about 60% of current lung cancer patients either never smoked or quit years ago. Who is really to blame here? Is it the addicts and former addicts or a society that allowed tobacco companies to sell their product without regulation?

Lung cancer advocates like me have gotten together and are trying to do something about fighting the stigma of lung cancer. We feel that supportive care and sympathy (not blame) is particularly important to patients living with lung cancer. Lung cancer patients have feelings of guilt and are isolated by an unspoken stigma associated with their diagnosis.

The stigma does more than just blame smokers. It pushes the responsibility of the disease away from society where it belongs and onto the patients and their families, where it shames them into silence. Their silence leads to the marked underfunding for the early detection and treatment of lung cancer.

I am not ashamed to have lung cancer. I am a victim, like many of the 70 million former smokers, who were addicted to tobacco and finally quit. And I am fighting for all of the former smokers who may eventually develop lung cancer. There needs to be an accepted screening protocol to detect lung cancer. That effort has the potential to save millions of lives.

Scanxiety

I had my quarterly PET/CT scans today. Since being diagnosed I have had these scans and blood tests done every three months, looking for evidence of cancer. To date, I have gotten through the exams with nothing but good news. The four little words I want to hear each time is we find "no evidence of disease." It doesn't mean you are cured. It means that there is nothing obvious going on that the doctors can detect. The disease is ALWAYS there, lurking. You are never cured. Cancer patients live with the disease and hope and pray to keep it at bay.

You become somewhat fatalistic, steeling yourself for bad news each time. You hope and pray for good news knowing deep down that one day the news may not be so good. Yes, people can live for many years with cancer, and you hope to be one of them. That does not stop you, however, from becoming anxious around scan time. I call it "scanxiety."

In the past two years I must have had close to a dozen scans. At first I was not bothered by the PET/CT (and could not understand people who are) until a scan I had in January of 2008.

The procedure involves the imaging center prepping you by injecting a radioactive isotope, which needs to circulate in your body for about an hour. After that, you are taken to the PET/CT machine. The CT scan is a relatively quick procedure and maybe takes 5 minutes. The full body PET scan, however, takes about 25 minutes normally, for someone my size.

For lung cancer, the technicians position you on a table with your arms above your head and strap you down to keep you from moving. You are told to "stay still and don't move". The technicians then leave the room and the lights are dimmed. The machine starts up with a soft whirring noise and the table slowly slides you into the tube head first.

You would think, what's the big deal? But those 25 minutes in the machine, with nothing but white walls of the tube surrounding you were the longest 25 minutes of my life, the first time I did it. The second time I did it in January of 2008 I was already apprehensive about the scan. That day the radiology center was having trouble with newly installed software that runs the machine. The computer kept crashing so the scan took nearly an hour. Toward the end I felt like I was being tortured. My fingers were numb and I became increasingly restless and panicky. The best way I can think to describe it is the feeling of slowly drowning and becoming increasingly more desperate to reach the surface. I was never so happy when that interminable test finally finished

Ever since, I have to have a sedative with my radio isotope injection to get me in a relaxed state. Yoko comes with me to hold my hand and stimulate me during the test. I also bring my i-pod along as a way of measuring the time and having something other than the walls of the machine to focus on. These days I am getting through the scans more easily and my anxiety is less than it was. Now let's hope and pray the results continue to be good.

Waiting on the test results is even worse than the test.

Reaching Milestones

When I was first diagnosed with lung cancer in late 2007, Yoko and I went to see my daughter Jessica in Tallahassee. She was then a first year freshman at Florida State. At the time, I really did not think I would live to see her graduate from college. Now, two years later, she is finishing her first semester as a junior. Next year at this time she'll be a senior and I will be one step closer to seeing all of my girls finish their undergraduate degrees.

When you have cancer you begin living your life with mental goals or milestones. In the early days you are just trying to get through treatments and live. If you are lucky enough to come out on the other side, like me, you begin to set goals for yourself. My first goal was to live long enough to see Paula married. Then I wanted to be well enough to take a once in a lifetime trip. (Yoko and I took a luxury three-week tour of Italy last year.) Now I want to live long enough to see Jessica graduate from college.

I have other things on my "bucket list" I would like to do. For example, I use to be a fairly accomplished horseman (dressage and show jumping); I always dreamed it would be fun go horseback riding on the open plains of Mongolia. I actually made it to Harbin, Manchuria one year on business but never made it to Mongolia. It's one of a number of countries in Asia I have not visited and would like to see one day.

As it so happens, Rotary District 6960 is organizing a Group Study Exchange (GSE) with a district in Eastern Siberia in May of 2010, just six months from now. It is a five week trip to Russia that I would love to make. As you might imagine, there is a lot of preparation to go on a trip like this. The GSE group trains together for about six months. Being an East Asian scholar of sorts I was thinking of volunteering to lead the GSE team to Siberia and afterward take a week to go riding in Mongolia. This is definitely a trip I would have to do alone (Yoko wants no part of this dream), but what an adventure would be! There's only one problem. I am not scheduled for another Pet/CT until April, 2010. What if I discover cancer on my next scan?

Changing gears for just a second… Last week our community lost another dear friend and a man with a heart of gold, Bill Van Dyk, to cancer. Bill was in the 2004 Leadership Charlotte Class with me and had won his battle with cancer years ago. He never made much of his original cancer diagnosis and you would not have known he had a recurrence until recently. He fought hard and I was somewhat dismayed at how rapidly he declined once the cancer spread. My heart goes out to his wife and family this holiday season. I think to myself, there but for the grace of God go I.

Cancer patients in remission are conscious of the fact that the beast can return at any time. For lung cancer patients, it is not just possible — it is probable. I for one wake up every day conscious of the fact that the clock is ticking. Time passes quickly and there is no time to waste.

Tomorrow I have an appointment to see Dr. John about removing my port. I have had the port for two years and it is a constant reminder of my cancer diagnosis. While I am at it, I am going to schedule a colonoscopy, which I should have done years ago. After that I will decide whether a trip to Siberia or horseback riding in Mongolia is in the cards. Let's hope!

Holiday Memories

I've always found it difficult to get into the holiday spirit living in Florida. Warm weather is somehow just not conducive to the joy of the holiday season.

I suppose the reason has to do with growing up in cold weather climates when I was a kid. I remember the years my family lived in Syracuse, New York. We had a snow-covered Christmas every year. Our house had a plate glass window in the living room on the second floor overlooking the front yard and street below. Our Christmas tree would be set near the living room window for all to see. On Christmas Eve the neighbors would line the street with brown paper bags weighted with sand to holding small candles. The candles were lit after dark and the street, lined on both sides with these glowing bags, would look like a runway landing. I remember taking in this scene standing at our living room window, scanning the sky for Santa's sleigh. There was house to house caroling on Christmas Eve and I remember one year Santa rode through the neighborhood on a fire truck throwing candy to the children who came out in the snow to greet him. That was a very special time and I think it is the reason the weather has to be cold for me to recall the excitement of childhood in the Christmas season.

After Syracuse, we moved to Pennsylvania and Christmas was never quite the same. By that time I was no longer looking to the sky for Santa, I was scouring the closets to see what was hidden beneath the coats. A white Christmas was a rarity in Horsham, PA. We had neighbors, Harry and Beryl Davis, who were obsessed with decorating their house at Christmas. I remember the living room tree was an artificial, all white tree decorated with red ornaments. They collected Christmas decorations and, in their den, they constructed an elaborate miniature Bavarian mountain village underneath a real tree with a toy train set running though it, tunnels and all. We always had fun with the Davis family at Christmas and New Years. To this day I exchange Christmas cards with Harry and Beryl, even though I have not seen them in 30 years.

After my time in PA, I moved farther south to Washington D.C., where I attended George Washington University. I joined the school chorus as a freshman and learned to sing Handel's Messiah for our annual Christmas concert. That first year we put on a joint production with Georgetown, American and Catholic University. It was an event attended by the Washington glitterati in formal attire. The venue was a Gothic chapel on the Georgetown Campus. It was a magical night when 200 student voices came together with the symphony to sing the Messiah to this crowd. To this day it does not feel like Christmas to me without hearing a live performance of the Messiah. When I do hear it, I get choked up. To me that glorious music is the voice of God.

The most idyllic Christmas I ever spent was in Jackson Hole when my kids were still little. I remember taking Paula and June to pick out a Christmas tree in the national forest and then dragging the tree (and the kids) down a mountain through the woods in waist-high snow. (That part was not fun for any of us!) We had a place that looked out to the Grand Tetons and we put up the freshly cut tree in the living room, near a stone fireplace. That Christmas I took a snowmobile ride through Yellowstone National Park in minus 40 degree weather, from the South Entrance to Ole Faithful, roughly 120 miles round trip. It was a picture postcard winter wonderland that I will never ever forget.

Christmas in Florida does not compare. Still, I'm glad to be alive and here to enjoy yet another Christmas. Next year maybe we'll go somewhere cold?

Keeping in Touch

My favorite part of Christmas is getting carefully crafted letters from old friends and acquaintances. One of my life-long friends, Eric Madsen, sends out a hilarious Christmas missive every year highlighting the antics of his (now grown) children. We generally don't hear much from Eric and his family during the year, but we never lose track of what is going on with the Madsen family thanks to Eric's annual Christmas letters.

Last year Eric wrote about how his boys "once hung on his every word and now hang him with every word." In the old days, he says, "he served as a fount of advice" for his children. Now any suggestion he makes is "met with rolling eyes, heaving sighs and cries of "ole school!"" Eric writes with a wink: "They are not as smart as they think. I'm still lucid enough to have them removed from my will. That's how we roll in my ole school!"

Those of us with children over the age of 18 can easily relate. At one point in my life I was teaching my three daughters — to put it delicately — the basics of good hygiene. Somewhere along the way our roles got reversed. Whatever happened to the wisdom of age? In a fast changing technological world it would seem, the older you get, the less you know.

I don't want to become obsolete before my time, so I made a concerted effort this year to try and keep up and not be too "ole school". For example, I asked my daughter Jessica to upload her music to my i-pod so I can learn what music kids are listening to these days. Still, I wouldn't know Taylor Swift if you put her in a photo line-up. I would have to go to class to learn all the pop culture trivia my kids seem to know naturally. Popular culture was never my strong suit, even when I was a kid.

Every year I feel I am falling still further behind. I only recently heard about the movie that's all the teenage rage — Twilight and New Moon. The entire country was going nuts about the sequel before I even knew it was a bestselling book and hit movie. I would not have known about any of it were it not for a news report on CNBC about the box office take! I guess we are what we read or listen to.

In my quest to stay current, about six months ago I decided to register on Facebook, because I was curious about how these social networking sites work. Suddenly I have 71 "friends" (many are people I knew in high school — more like acquaintances than "friends" really.) Nevertheless, my "friends" post something about their day, every day. And if that is not enough, I can follow them on Twitter and learn about their every passing thought or emotion. Do I really want to know that much about them? No, I don't think so. (And I'm quite sure they really don't know (or care to know) that much about me.)

My daughter June, on the other hand, is someone I DO care about and she sends me mostly nonsensical "tweets" on a regular basis. I love to get these inane blurbs, but half the time I have no idea what she is talking about. For example, the latest tweet she sent was "Hello Wednesday. I thought you were Friday."(She sends news flashes like this at 9 PM Hawaiian time, causing my cell phone to alert for an incoming message at 3 AM.) Huh? Hello? I tweet back: "Forget about what day it is…what planet are you on? Love Dad. "

Keeping in touch is an act of love…or at least it use to be. But with all the "communicating" going on these days — through cell phones, texting, e-mailing, social networks and the like — what is there left to say of substance in a Christmas card or letter? It may be "ole school" but I still love getting a Christmas card or letter with a hand written note from people you really know and love.

May God bless us all with love, happiness, peace, good health and prosperity! Now, let's go make 2010 another unforgettable year!

Part IV — 2010

A Preview of 2010

I've been thinking about 2010 and what the year will bring. First I have to say I am glad to be here to live another year. I never forget that every day is a blessing. Someone sent me an electronic Christmas card that had a quote from Winston Churchill that said, "We make a living by what we get, we make a life by what we give." How true that is.

The year 2009 has been a hard year for most people. The economy has been in a slump and families are hurting. During the year I became Chairman of the Board of the Virginia B Andes Volunteer Community Clinic, which saw more than 4,500 patients in need. The clinic provides urgent or episodic care for folks in Charlotte County who don't have or can't afford health insurance. It's an alternative to going to the emergency room. I can't tell you how proud I am of the work we do at the free clinic and pharmacy. We have received fantastic support from the community at large and the medical community in particular. Helping to organize and fund the clinic is truly one of the best things I have ever done in my life. I am looking forward to continuing to work for the clinic in the New Year.

In April I attended the National Lung Cancer Partnership Advocate Summit in Dallas, which gave me the idea of organizing the Free to Breathe 5K event in October. I've developed a passion about doing something about cancer and lung cancer in particular thanks to the inspired leadership of this organization. Not a day goes by that I don't think about cancer and how quickly lives are taken by this disease. I lost a number of friends and clients — two to lung cancer — during the year. We are already planning the next Free to Breathe 5K event for November 13th 2010 at Charlotte Sports Park.

In the New Year I am serving as honorary chair of the Port Charlotte Relay for Life, to benefit our local chapter of the American Cancer Society.

Yoko and I have never been in the habit of planning travel far in advance, but with the girls out of the house and on their own, it is hard to get together without some forethought. We are already making plans for the New Year.

I am expecting my Mom to come down from Pennsylvania for a few weeks in January and I am also hoping to see other friends and relatives over the course of the winter. January is shaping up to be a busy month.

In February Yoko wants to go to Tallahassee to attend "Dance Marathon." Since her freshman year my daughter Jessica has been involved in organizing this fundraiser to benefit Shands Children's Hospital in Gainesville. We want to give Jessie our support on Valentine's Day. I also want to make a trip to Scottsdale, Arizona, to play golf, if we can find the time.

If all is well, this summer I would like to take a trip to the mountains of Tennessee with Yoko and the dog. The plan would be to rent a cabin and spend a few months of the summer working from a cool mountain retreat. (I would have remote access to my workstation.) I have a book project to work on and a screen play I would like to finally finish as well.

This time next year, if all goes well, I am planning to rent a condo somewhere in Colorado for a week of skiing and winter fun with the family. All the girls have promised to be there. Now that is something to look forward to in 2010!

Lung Cancer Patient's Feelings of Guilt

If you read the "Feeling Fit" section of the Charlotte Sun, you'll notice that it is teeming with announcements for all kinds of support groups meetings. It seems like nearly every malady imaginable is covered, so it was surprising to me that Charlotte County had no lung cancer support group.

Thanks to the effort of my friends Irene and Carlos, that is no longer true. The first meeting of the Charlotte County Lung Cancer Support Group was held in December, with about 18 people in attendance. Many who came are lung cancer patients, but there were others who are caregivers grieving for a recently lost loved one. The group plans to get together once a month on the second Tuesday.

Having a support group is invaluable. No one knows better the range of emotions you have after a lung cancer diagnosis than another patient. Sharing those feeling is important therapy. Since there was no support group in the area when I was diagnosed, I went on the Internet to seek out support and information. The first thing I did was purchase books on lung cancer. I also found an online support group, hosted by the Lung Cancer Alliance. This group provides a resource to the experiences of thousands of lung cancer patients and caregivers. (See http://www.inspire.com/groups/lung-cancer-alliance-survivors/)

One of the best books I found is called "Lung Cancer — Myths, Facts, Choices and Hope" written by famed lung cancer researcher Dr. Claudia Henschke and Peggy McCarthy, founder of the Alliance for Lung Cancer Advocacy. I read the 400 pages cover to cover in a day, devouring the content as if my life depended on it. What I learned in those pages, in fact, helped save my life. Knowing that people do survive a lung cancer diagnosis provided me the motivation to fight and to believe that there was a way through to a new chapter in my life.

The sad fact is that many lung cancer patients have an overwhelming sense of guilt. They feel responsible, somehow, for contracting the disease. Many lung cancer patients adopt the attitude that they "deserve what they get" and choose to get no treatment. These feelings of guilt may be reinforced by family, friends, and even healthcare providers, who Peggy McCarthy says "view lung cancer as a lesson in the wages of sin." "Pervasive negative feelings about smoking", she says, results in "lung cancer patients not being offered aggressive life-saving treatments." Guilt ridden patients frequently don't demand treatments that could prolong or improve their lives. McCarthy says we need to confront these attitudes and change them. I agree. The attitude of some in the medical community is particularly irksome.

There is an interesting story in the book talking about Alice Steward Trillen, who at the age of 38, coughed up a small clot of blood, went for an X-ray, and learned she had lung cancer. The book quotes Trillen as saying "I was young. I was healthy. I never smoked a cigarette in my life. The doctors tried to give me explanations for the tumor and seemed embarrassed that they couldn't come up with any. I sneaked a look at my hospital chart and found in one doctor's report on me the phrase, "Patient gives the story that she never smoked." This doctor simply found it necessary to blame me for having lung cancer."

Lung cancer patients need support and encouragement from their family, friends and doctors if they are going to beat the disease. Feelings of guilt and remorse and assigning blame for the disease only make recovery more difficult.

Irene and Carlos may not realize it, but I have no doubt the support group they have formed is going to help save or extend lives. I plan to attend every month.

Helping Our Community

I joined the board of the St. Vincent DePaul Community Pharmacy about four years ago. That entity has since morphed into St. Vincent DePaul Community Healthcare Inc., now doing business as The Virginia B. Andes Volunteer Community Clinic. I served on the board beginning in 2005 and became treasurer in 2007.

That year the board decided to expand the mission from providing life-saving prescription drugs to also providing urgent and episodic care to the working poor and uninsured in Charlotte County. Charlotte County is ranked 15th among 67 counties in Florida with residents without healthcare. We also have one of the highest unemployment rates in the state.

The original idea for the clinic was to relieve our congested hospital emergency rooms, which are required by law to treat anyone with illness or injury, whether they can pay or not. Emergency room costs are estimated to be six times more than treatment in a physicians' office. Without our clinic, the emergency room was the only after-hours option to access healthcare for the poor.

I was diagnosed with lung cancer in October 2007, at about the time the board decided to go forward with opening the clinic. Everything seemed to miraculously come together. We were able to get an ideal location near Fawcett and Peace River Hospital on county land at the Family Services Center. All three area-hospitals — Fawcett, Peace River and Charlotte Regional — provided us with seed money to bring in and set up a modular clinic on the site. As treasurer, I was responsible for funding this undertaking. My thought had always been that if the area hospitals and the community at large fully supported the effort, we could make it work.

In fact the clinic has been a win-win for everyone involved. Since opening in February of 2008, we have seen more than 9,000 patients and have dispensed thousands of prescription drugs to those in need. Treating patients (for high blood pressure, flu, diabetes, etc) who might otherwise go untreated is helping to keep them out of the hospital with a more serious disease (heart attack, stroke, pneumonia). I believe what we are doing at the clinic is what Christ intended for us to do on earth, and may be one reason God is letting me live. He wants me to help keep His good work going.

In 2008 I became President of the clinic and, under the leadership of Suzanne Roberts, our executive director, we have found our feet and we are moving forward with wide ranging health services. Today we have more than 180 volunteers, including physicians, nurses, and pharmacists who provide their time and expertise to help our patients. We would be nowhere without them.

In the first year of operation, Virginia B. Andes, a longtime community volunteer, provided the clinic with vitally needed operating dollars. Without her support we might have had to close our doors for lack of funding. Despite the generous funding we receive from the area hospitals, the county government and United Way, operating a free clinic is expensive. Our bare bones budget this year, which is based on known sources of income, is roughly $300,000. That amount allows us to operate at a subsistence level, but we are severely constrained on what we are able to do. We have set a goal to raise another $100,000 in operating dollars from the community this year.

When Are You" Cured"?

I went to the January Lung Cancer Support Group meeting this week. The meeting had 28 people in attendance and our speaker was Dr. Tom, a local thoracic surgeon. Dr. Tom's presentation and the medical discussion that ensued made me once again realize how little I know about cancer and how much there is to learn. The discussion was wide ranging but there was one question that came up that I thought was kind of interesting. One of the members of the group asked…is there a cure for lung cancer?

Since being diagnosed, not a day has gone by that I don't think about having cancer. It is always with me and on my mind. I am living my life today as if there is nothing wrong. I'm in a clinical trial and go for shots every six weeks. Other than that, I am not being treated for cancer any longer. Am I "cured?" Well, if I am not dead and the disease is nowhere to be found, I guess you could say I am "cured". Will it last? That is an entirely different matter.

Until you have lived five years after a cancer diagnosis, you are a cancer patient. If you make it to five years, in the medical world, you are considered a "survivor." If you die from cancer at any time you are a cancer victim. I am almost half way to becoming a rare lung cancer "survivor" because I have lived two and a half years since my diagnosis. The fact of the matter is that you are never really "cured" of cancer, even if you "survive" for a while.

If you are asymptomatic, that does not mean that there are no active cancer cells running around in your body. Dr. Tom had a useful analogy to explain the concept of a false negative when thinking about test results: if a mouse in the room is spotted running across the floor it is positive affirmation there is a mouse in the room. We can see the mouse. But if we don't see a mouse, does it mean there is none in the room?

We can never know if we are ever "cancer free." My current status is NED — no evidence of disease. What they mean by that is that they can't find it, but since I had it, we can't say that it is no longer there. The best we can say is that there is no EVIDENCE that it is there. We don't see the mouse any longer.

The cruel thing about cancer is that you can be easily lulled into the belief that you are cured. You are living your normal life after treatment, going along your merry way…and then…. BOOM… the other shoe drops and you find you have a nodule or tumor where there was none before. All cancer patients in remission live with the fear that cancer could turn your life upside down at any time. Still, the longer you are in remission the more hopeful you become about the future.

Speaking of the future, I have a three year lease on an Acura that ends in February. I have been thinking about what my next car should be and whether I should buy the next car or lease it. Yoko and I debated a lot of choices. Ultimately we decided to buy. Since this might be the last car I ever purchase…why not get something really memorable. What I selected is a completely impractical Mercedes roadster convertible. You can't even get a set of golf clubs in it when the roof is down, but I love it! Now all I have to do is come up with something appropriate for a license plate… Maybe "IM CURED" would fit the ticket?

Changing Culture

Yoko and I were watching the AFC and NFC Championship games on Sunday. She has really learned to enjoy American football and gets as excited watching a game as anyone I know. She has also become pretty knowledgeable about the rules of the game and the players. For example, she knew Percy Harvin, who now plays for Minnesota used to be a Florida Gator. One of her favorite teams is Boise State. (She fell in love with them after their unbelievable victory over Oklahoma at the Fiesta Bowl in 2007.)

Yoko generally likes college football better than professional football. I think her preference for college football has something to do with the purity of amateur athletics and the fun and raw emotion displayed by young and enthusiastic fans. Anyway, football is a part of American culture that Yoko admires.

Baseball is the Japanese national pastime — but Japanese baseball is different from what we play here in America. There is a very funny book call "The Chrysanthemum and the Bat", written by a friend of mine, Robert Whiting, which describes the subtle cultural differences in how baseball is practiced and played in Japan. The book's title is a humorous allusion to Ruth Benedict's classic, "The Chrysanthemum and the Sword", a serious anthropological study of Japanese culture commissioned by the US Government during the Second World War. The theme of Whiting's book is that Japanese culture imbues and colors every aspect of life in Japan, including something as mundane as baseball.

Yoko and I talk about "American culture verses Japanese culture" on a regular basis. The discussion is usually triggered by something I bring home from the store (unhealthy snacks), something on television (Viagra commercials during family viewing hours or personal injury attorneys advertising for victims), or something that she observes in my interactions with other people. (I'm frequently accused by my wife of having done or said something that is ill mannered, impolite, or inconsiderate.)

What triggered tonight's discussion was a new Wal-Mart commercial aired during the football games. A dad, dressed as a clown, jumps into a room where children are playing at a birthday party and stubs his foot on a child's toy. He screams at the top of his lungs and scares the kids away, ruining the party. Yoko understands that this is intended to be humorous, but she doesn't think it is funny. She thinks it is rather violent and unappealing. I can't disagree.

Yoko objects to "reality" TV shows, like Donald Trump's "The Apprentice," that pit people against one another and challenges contestants to disparage and humiliate each other. Where, she wonders, is the human kindness and Christian values of love and compassion we espouse? She dislikes reality TV in general, which she sees as "mean" spirited and has none of the fun or innocence of Alan Funt's "Candid Camera" or America's Funniest Home Videos, which she likes. Japanese love slapstick and other forms of humor, but most often Japanese are self-deprecating. Entertainment and joking is seldom directed at someone else's expense.

I've been reading a book by the brilliant Charles Munger, Warren Buffett's acclaimed business partner, called "On Success." Munger writes about the psychology of human misjudgment and addresses the issue of excessive self-regard tendency. (For example, 90% of Swedish drivers judge themselves to be above average.) Yoko believes that Americans in general suffer from high self-regard and self-centeredness. That might be true for the Japanese as well. I agree with a lot of what Yoko thinks about American culture, but I sometimes wonder if she realizes that she is seeing American culture through her own cultural filter. No doubt there is a lot that we Americans could learn from the Japanese.

Munger writes that "Man's excess self-regard typically makes him prefer people like himself." Munger concludes that we need to be objective in making assessments about self, family, friends and property to avoid the folly of high self-regard. It's a good lesson for all of us.

Handling Bad News

Let's face it. This has not been a great ten years. The Internet bubble burst in 2000. Accounting scandals ended in the bankruptcy of Enron and WorldCom and the destruction of my former employer, Arthur Andersen. We endured 9/11 and the collapse of the World Trade Center in 2001, the onset of war in Afghanistan and Iraq in 2002. The year 2004 brought hurricanes to Florida and a tidal wave that devastated Indonesia and Thailand. Katrina and the disaster in New Orleans followed in 2005.

Today we are experiencing the aftermath of falling real estate values, the Madoff swindle, and the near collapse of our financial markets. We are dealing with a severe recession, high unemployment and a devastating disaster in Haiti. When will the bad news end?

When things go wrong it's important to look for the silver lining. As bad as things are, life can always be worse. Ask any Haitian.

Erma Bombeck wrote a book called, "If Life is a Bowl of Cherries, What am I Doing in the Pits?" Well, guess it depends on how you look at things. Sometimes being in the pits is a plus! I became a stock broker in 1999 and was only starting to build my book of business when the tech bubble ended and stock prices collapsed. I didn't have a lot of clients that got hurt because I didn't have a lot of clients! The silver lining for me was that there were a lot of unhappy investors out there. That fact and a positive outlook provided me with the opportunity to gain a foothold in the market as a financial advisor. While established brokers were avoiding calls from clients, I was knocking on the door. You could say starting my career in a down market was kind of a lucky break.

Cancer patients deal with bad news and disappointment on a regular basis. It comes with the territory. The first bad news is the diagnosis itself. Then you learn if it is operable or not. Is it in the lymph nodes? Has it spread? Is there more than one tumor? Are the drug treatments working? Can you be cured? Will you still be able to work? Will your insurance pay for all the treatments you need? The list goes on and on. Where's cancer's silver lining? I have to say that cancer has helped me appreciate my family and friends and the blessings I have. I am much more keenly aware of my mortality and the limited time I have on earth. I have finally gotten my priorities straight and am trying to accomplish all that I would hope to do with my life. I think cancer has made me a better person and has improved the quality of my life.

I've been reading about the life of someone named David Welch, who, at the age of 38, was diagnosed with brain cancer. David passed away a year ago, but he created a website called 38Lemon (named after the age he was diagnosed with a tumor the size of a lemon). David's journal is inspirational reading for anyone with cancer. He lived for four years 35 days from his date of diagnosis and wrote about his life and treatment nearly every day until the day he died. He was an accomplished musician, a successful entrepreneur, a writer and an artist. He had family and friends who loved him. He was courageous in facing his disease and passionate about not giving up on life. He is truly someone who knew how to turn lemons into lemonade.

Yoko and I have had our share of personal tragedy and heartache, but we have come through it all. I think we go through life, especially when we are young, pretending nothing bad can happen. When it does, we are devastated. Maybe we should just expect bad news — like biting into a cherry with a pit — and just be happy we don't break a tooth. Focus on the fact that life is sweet and savor the moment.

Feeling the Love on Valentine's Day

Yoko and I took off for Tallahassee on Valentine's Day weekend to see our daughter Jessica at Florida State. Jessie is deeply involved with Dance Marathon, which is a 40-hour danceathon to raise money for The Children's Miracle Network (CMN). Last year FSU's Dance Marathon donated more than $380,000 in proceeds to Shands Children Hospital in Gainesville, a CMN supported facility.

Jessie has volunteered to help with the FSU event for the past three years. She serves on the Dance Marathon organizing committee and is responsible for media production, including creating and editing all the music, video and still photography used prior to, during and after the event. Dance Marathon has become the centerpiece of her college career. In fact, because of Dance Marathon, Jessie has decided to pursue event management as a career.

My alma mater, Penn State, is the school that came up with the idea of a Dance Marathon fundraiser. It was started in 1973 by the Penn State's Inter-fraternity Council. That year just $2,000 was raised by 39 couples dancing for 30 hours straight. Penn State donated the money it raised to the Butler County Association of Retarded Citizens.

In 1977, Dance Marathon was changed to a 48-hour event and became an annual benefit for the Four Diamonds Fund at Penn State's Hershey Medical Center. In 1990, Indiana University began their own Dance Marathon to raise funds for the Ryan White Infectious Disease Center at Riley Hospital for Children.

In 1995, the Children's Miracle Network developed a fundraising program inspired by these early dance marathons. The first year of the program, four schools participated and raised a total of $142,000. Six more schools, including FSU, were added to the program the following year, raising $300,000. And the rest, as they say, is history.

Today, across the nation, more than 80 schools hold Dance Marathons to raise money for Children's Miracle Network. The FSU Dance Marathon alone has raised $2.2 million since 1996. More than $40 million has been raised across the nation since 1996. What a great story!

Yoko and I decided this year would be a good time to check out what Jessie has been up to all this time, so we made plans to go up on Valentine's Day weekend to witness the event for ourselves. After that we were going to continue on to Blue Ridge, Georgia for a romantic weekend and look for a summer cabin.

I wasn't sure what to expect when we showed up at the Leon Civic Center to witness the opening of Dance Marathon. Throbbing music with a heavy drumbeat was blaring as we made our way into the heavily decorated hall where all the dancing was about to begin. In years gone by the FSU marathon was one session that continued for 36 hours straight. This year to increase participation (and the amount of money raised) the kids decided to do two sessions of 20 hours each with a three hour break in between. (600 kids participate in each session.) We got there just at the kids were entering the hall for the second session.

The excitement in the hall was tangible as the dancers got ready to stand and dance for 20 consecutive hours. The kickoff started with a 34-minute music video countdown, largely edited by my daughter. Then at exactly 7 PM the marathon officially begins. The organizing committee starts things off with a high energy nine minute line dance that all 1200 dancers will learn before the end of the night. (The line dance happens at the top of each hour for the entire 20 hours.

You could feel the love of the student dancers literally giving of themselves on Valentine's Day. The marathon, which ended at 3 PM on Sunday brought in more than $ 450,000. Yoko and I could not be more proud of the part Jessie played.

Anger about Government Indifference

Back in November I wrote an online post about how lung cancer patients need to fight the stigma of lung cancer. It is a topic that really hit home with lung cancer patients and I have ignited a little firestorm of discussion and debate on the topic. Lung cancer patients are angry with the government's indifference.

My original posting really had everything to do with discussing how to fight the stigma of lung cancer and nothing to do with the negative health effects of smoking. Smoking is bad for you. There is no debate any longer and that was not the point of my posting. Yet it seems whenever I talk about lung cancer I end up in a discussion about smoking. It's infuriating because that is exactly my point! It's not about smoking. It's about lung cancer — how to detect it, treat it and prevent it!

Remember the 1980's and the AIDS movement? I think that lung cancer has the same kind of stigma attached to it. There was little funding for AIDS research in the early 1980's because AIDS was thought to be caused by the "lifestyle" of gays and drug addicts. In the same way, lung cancer today has only a small amount of research funding because the disease is thought to be a self-inflicted "lifestyle" disease caused by smoking. AIDS got more attention and research dollars when activists marched on Washington and people began to realize that "innocents" (i.e. mothers and newborns) were also getting the disease.

I think lung cancer patients need to be pointing out two things: not only do many innocent non-smokers develop lung cancer, but people who QUIT smoking, even decades ago and live a healthy lifestyle today, can and do frequently develop lung cancer.

More dollars devoted to research into lung cancer early detection could save 70,000 lives a YEAR, according to an actuarial study released on February 16 by Lung Cancer Alliance. If nothing else, we should be fighting to give FUTURE lung cancer patients a better chance of surviving the disease. There are 70 million former smokers at risk in this country and many more millions who were or are exposed to second hand smoke (and other lung cancer causing agents). They need to be given a chance. They shouldn't just be written off with our "oh well, deserves you right" attitude.

My interest is to find a way to increase public understanding for the critical need for lung cancer research. We need to fight the stigma of lung cancer with facts.

The legal sale of cigarettes continues to this day despite the fact that nicotine is KNOWN to create a habit forming addiction that can kill or harm you just as surely as lead-based paint or asbestos. Where is the government in regulating THIS drug and keeping it out of the hands of our children? Where is the Consumer Products Safety Commission?

I am on a drug-trial for Stimuvax — a lung cancer vaccine that could save or extend the lives of all of us struggling with lung cancer, but the law requires extensive trials and testing before allowing a new drug on the market. (I'd like to see the trials the Federal government did on cigarettes (and other carcinogens) before allowing them on the market!) Shouldn't we be giving a drug like Stimuvax to people at high risk of developing lung cancer? Don't the tens of millions of people at risk of developing lung cancer deserve research into early detection or, better yet, potential "lung cancer preventatives" especially since it is not likely we will ever ban the sale of tobacco products?

In the next five years 800,000 people in this country will die from lung cancer before potential lifesaving drugs like Stimuvax are approved for use. What, on earth, is the FDA protecting us from?

Trip to the Panhandle

After Dance Marathon on Valentine's Day Yoko and I planned to head north to Blue Ridge, Georgia to check out mountain cabins for the summer months. The weekend turned out to be unusually cold. The forecast for Georgia was snow and ice in the mountains where we were headed. In fact, travel conditions were so bad our real estate agent called to advise us NOT to come!

We had planned to leave Tallahassee for Georgia Sunday afternoon but now, suddenly, we had no place to go. We had never seen any of the Florida panhandle, so this was a good opportunity to explore. We decided to go west as far as the Destin/ Fort Walton Beach area and then take two days to drive home along the coast, browsing for real estate along the way.

We found a "four star" Hilton Hotel online that looked to be quite nice for a reasonable price. The off-season rate advertised on the Internet was $109 per night. We figured we would not need reservations at this time of year anyway, so we left Tallahassee around 4 PM Sunday and made it to the Sandestin Hilton by dusk.

When we arrived there was no bellman or valet on duty to greet us and the lobby was deserted. I dropped Yoko off with the bags and self parked. When we got to the front desk, Olga, the receptionist, greeted us with a dour demeanor. I asked if there were any rooms available. In a Slavic accent Olga said there were "only a few rooms" available at $169 per night. Huh? Who does she think she's kidding? I don't think there were 10 cars in the parking lot I had just come from and not a soul was in sight.

I explained to Olga that I had checked the Internet before selecting the Hilton and the partial ocean view room rate advertised was $109 per night. Olga explained that that was the internet reservation rate, not the walk-in rate. "Oh," I said, "Should I just go back to my car and make a reservation on my laptop at the $109.00 rate?" At that point, Olga relented and gave us a very nice room for $109.00. Then she informed us that there was a $10 charge for parking and $20 for valet parking. Hmmm…well, it's too late for the valet parking, I thought. "Is there someplace I can park where I do not get charged?" (Of course, I already knew the answer was "no.") Hilton has now earned my enmity along with the airlines that do a head fake with "low fares" and then charge for baggage and incidentals. I'll avoid Hilton Hotels in the future.

On Monday morning we checked out and drove along Route 98, which follows the panhandle coast. At times it seemed like we were the only car on the road. We stopped and visited a few of the newer developments along Emerald Coast Parkway, including an upscale development called Blue Mountain Beach, another one called Watermark, and St. Georges Island. Everywhere we went we found a plethora of "for sale" and "foreclosure" signs, exceedingly high prices, and no customers or tourists in sight.

We finally arrived in Perry, Florida, exhausted, hungry and needing to find a clean place to stay. Luckily, we came across a sparkling new Holiday Inn Express. I asked if there were rooms available and the smiling young desk clerk said we could have any room in the hotel for $99 a night. The price included a buffet breakfast and a newspaper in the morning. "Do you charge for parking?" I asked. She just laughed. I'm sure she thought I was joking. Without our asking, she offered to give us a $15 discount to $84 if we are members of AARP! Sold!

This is the first time I've ever been offered a senior discount. I'm glad to have lived long enough to have seen this day! Are you listening Hilton Hotels?

A Dose of Reality

I'm participating in a double-blind, Stage III study of a lung cancer vaccine. Every six weeks I drive just over 2 hours from Punta Gorda to New Port Richey to receive my injections. (Because it's a blind study, I don't know if I am getting the experimental drug or sugar water.) On my visit this past Monday I saw my study doctor, who exclaimed, "This drug must be working!" I said to the physician, "How can you know that? This is a double blind study. Neither you nor I know if I am getting the real deal or a placebo."

The study doctor admitted that he doesn't know for sure. But, he explained, it's highly unusual for someone to do as well as I appear to be doing, given my diagnosis. He naturally concluded that it must be the trial drug.

Then I asked him: "In your 30 year career as an oncologist, how many inoperable Stage IIIA lung cancer patients have you seen survive 5 years or more?" His answer was depressing. "Only one… and that woman survived just over five years after undergoing chemo nearly the entire time."

The conversation was a real downer for me. I should be encouraged by the fact I am doing so well relative to most lung cancer patients. But his comment about late stage lung cancer's low survival rate shocked me back into the reality of my diagnosis. Despite my healthy appearance, I face a low probability of being a long term survivor. The drug I am taking has been shown in previous trials to help extend life for one to three years, but it is not a cure. Eventually, the cancer returns. That reality hit me this week like a ton of bricks.

Until Monday I was thinking of myself as "cured". In fact, a few weeks ago I ordered a vanity license plate for my car that reads "IM CURED". Now I hope I haven't jinxed myself! My next CT/PET scan is in a few weeks. We'll see what the results bring.

This past December I elected to have my infusion port removed. It was an act of faith that I will not need more chemotherapy in the foreseeable future. It gave me a psychological lift to have that lump of metal out of my chest. I felt restored to my former self and more optimistic about the future.

The only other reminders that I have lung cancer have been my cloudy eyesight and the neuropathy in my feet and hands. I had my eyes checked a year ago and was shocked to learn that I have developed cataracts in both eyes. I did not know it at the time I was having treatments, but apparently the steroids used in chemotherapy can cause cataracts.

I noticed that my eyesight has gotten worse. I can hit a golf ball but I can't see it land. It's hard for me to read the computer screen at work and at night the glare of on-coming headlights has made it harder to see the road.

My vision has deteriorated to the point where I decided I need to do something about it. After consulting with my colleague from the community clinic, Dr. David Klein, I decided to go ahead with cataract surgery and take care of this problem now rather than wait. Were I to have a recurrence of cancer that requires chemotherapy, corrective eye surgery would most definitely be off the table.

On Thursday I went into the hospital to have the cataract in my right eye removed and an artificial lens implanted. I stayed home Friday to recover. That's three out of five days of work missed this week for health related issues. Worst of all, golf is out of the question this weekend.

I guess I should be grateful I'm doing so well!

Royal Rife's Amazing Cancer Discoveries

There are all sorts of treatments for cancer, but to date a "cancer cure" has not been found — or so I thought. In fact, we can't even agree on the cause or causes of cancer. One thing is for sure: treating cancer — whatever the cause — is big business and growing.

For some time now I have been reading about the history of cancer research, including Dr. Devra Davis' book "The Secret History of the War on Cancer" which focuses on environmental toxins and carcinogens. The theme of this book is that economic interests — not science — drives public health policy. The tobacco industry's 30-year campaign to undermine evidence linking cigarettes to lung cancer is but one example Davis cites. If cell phones were definitively proven to lead to brain tumors, do you think the cell phone industry would act any differently than the tobacco companies did?

Another book, "Toxic Treatments: Surviving the Cancer Wars" by Penelope Williams, speaks to how offshore alternative treatments, offered in places such as Bermuda and Mexico and often condemned as being scams operated by medical quacks, have, in fact, been started by dedicated cancer researchers who were formerly employed at some of the world's most prestigious cancer research centers. No doubt there are some medical quacks selling false hope to cancer patients. But surely some alternative treatments have merit, even if the science for why something works is not understood. Being unorthodox and working outside established medical dogma, however, looks to be a lousy career choice for cancer researchers.

One of my friends, who used to work as a consultant to the National Cancer Institute, explained to me how difficult it is to get cancer research funded unless the proposed research falls within the realm of known science and is already "practically proven".

I think by now anyone interested in cancer research has heard of John Kanzius, a Sanibel Island, Florida cancer patient who was experimenting with radio waves and nano particles to treat cancers of all sorts. Kanzius was featured on CBS's 60 Minutes in 2008 as the unlikely, self-taught medical-industry-outsider who just may have found a cure for cancer. The basic idea Kanzius came up with is to inject patients with metallic nano particles that attach to cancer cells and then heat the particles and destroy the cells using harmless radio waves. It's a breakthrough idea, but it is not exactly new.

Dr. Royal Rife acclaimed by his biographer as "one of the greatest scientific geniuses of the 20th century" was a respected microbiologist and physicist. Rife began researching a cure for cancer in 1920. By 1932 he had isolated a virus found in every form of cancer, called the BX virus, and learned how to destroy it with electromagnetic (radio) frequency waves (the way sound waves can destroy glass.)

Rife worked with the most respected researchers in America in that era. In 1934, a Special Research Committee at University of Southern California oversaw the laboratory research and cancer clinic that treated 16 terminally ill patients with Rife's frequency machine. All 16 patients in the famous 1934 clinic were "cured" of their cancer within months.

Follow-up clinics run by USC and independent physicians between 1935 and 1937 confirmed the results. So why has no one heard of Royal Rife and his fantastic cancer cure?

In the 1987 book called "The Rife Report" biographer, Barry Lynes, assigns primary blame to Morris Fishbein, alleged to be a shakedown artist who headed the all powerful American Medical Association from the mid-1920s until 1949.

When Fishbein's overtures to buy Rife's technology were turned away, Lynes alleges that Fishbein used his position to shut down Rife's company and discredit his reputation and research. It's a complex tale well worth reading.

Springtime for Health Care Reform

I have been an advocate of health care reform since moving back to the US from Japan. Universal health care is offered in Japan and it works. The downside is the astronomically high taxes it imposes and the resulting government debt. Japan's debt to gross domestic product has nearly reached 200% — the highest in the OECD. (Japan's sovereign debt is currently rated AA by S&P.)

As president of The Virginia B. Andes Volunteer Community Clinic, I know, first hand, how great the need is for access to affordable healthcare here in Charlotte County. Our estimate is that 20% to 30% of Charlotte County residents are uninsured and, as a result, don't see a doctor on a regular basis. When there is a medical issue, uninsured people are more likely to end up in the emergency room with a serious problem.

I am very proud of our clinic's role in trying to address this issue in our community. We can thank the 180 unpaid volunteers — doctors, nurses, pharmacists and laymen — who are on the front lines of this issue. These are neighbors helping neighbors. We operate our free clinic and pharmacy with one full time executive director, a part-time medical director, and two part time office staff.

This year our clinic and pharmacy will operate on a bare bones budget of just under $300,000. We expect to see 4,500 patients for urgent and episodic care and hand out 120 or more life saving prescriptions a week. Last year we logged more than 26,000 donated hours, with an estimated labor value of $1.6 million. For every dollar donated to the Virginia B Andes Volunteer Community Clinic, we are providing something on the order of $8 in benefit to the community, including the value of medical services, prescription medications, and reduced unreimbursed emergency room costs for local hospitals. That's a pretty good investment. In fact, I think it's a model for what we could be doing in every county in the country.

Unfortunately, for the last year, the health care debate has been about insurance, not about providing health care services to the poor. I'm sad to say there are no federal dollars to support America's 1200 existing volunteer clinics in the new law.

As a cancer patient, I am relieved that I am now able to obtain insurance and be treated, despite my pre-existing condition. But I would be just as happy if I could walk into any healthcare facility, like our clinic, and be taken care of without the need for insurance at all.

In the new bill, the government got rid of the banks as middlemen for student loans, saving $62 billion over the next 10 years. How much money would we save in the health care system without insurance middlemen? The free market in health care should be about health care providers competing with one another, not about competition between health care insurance carriers who, as far as I can tell, add no real value.

The doctors at the Virginia B. Andes Volunteer Community Clinic are protected under sovereign immunity from lawsuits arising from the care of our patients. Volunteers, who register to serve qualified uninsured (income less than 200% of Federal poverty level) without compensation, are protected by the State of Florida. Patients can sue, but recovery is limited to $100,000. It would be hard to find a lawyer willing to take on a medical malpractice case where the upside is so small.

I was disappointed the issue of tort reform wasn't addressed in the current legislation as I think it is another key to making healthcare affordable.

I have to say I am happy that something is being done about our broken healthcare system. I can't say I am happy with the solution or the cost of the new law. Let's hope the focus of the debate now shifts to providing quality healthcare at a reasonable cost.

Stressing Over Too Much to Do and Bad News

I must say as I write this I am feeling a little stressed. I have many things going on and many balls in the air. I feel one may drop and go "SPLAT" at any time. It has been a struggle for me to keep up with all I am committed to doing. As my sister Jane likes to say, "I'm busier than a one armed paper hanger."

To try and manage my time, I decided to replace my simple cell phone with a Blackberry. Having this kind of device is a two edged sword. I may have a better handle on what's on the calendar, but in the age of instant communication, I feel inundated with messages and reminders about all of my commitments and doctor appointments.

Here is what my week has been like.

I had cataract surgery on my right eye a few weeks ago. On Monday morning, before work, I saw Dr. Klein for follow-up. He says he is going to need to make some adjustments. I can definitely see more clearly out of my right eye, but my vision is out of focus. I understand it takes a few months to fully heal. I have another appointment in a few weeks for more follow-up. In the meantime, Moe, my dog, ate the eye patch I was to use when I sleep.

On Tuesday I had an appointment to see my primary care doctor, who examined an infected cyst on my back. I got a prescription for Cipro (an antibiotic) and another follow-up appointment in a few weeks.

I had my CT/Pet Scan two weeks ago and I saw Dr. Scott to review the results on Thursday. My scans were clear and I continue to show no evidence of disease. (Thank you, Jesus!) My CEA levels — a blood marker for cancer — are in the normal range. You could not ask for a better outcome. We agreed that my next scans should be in June. If I am clear in three months, we'll change to six month intervals between scans.

I told Dr Scott about seeing my primary care doctor to look at a cyst on my back. (Dr. Scott knew I had an infection as it showed up in the scan.) Dr. Scott also examined my back and agreed that what I have is probably a sebaceous cyst. In all likelihood it is NOT cancerous. Nevertheless, in an abundance of caution, he sent me to see a general surgeon. Next week, after the infection is cleared up, I'll have the cyst removed and examined.

After seeing Dr. Scott I literally had to run to the Virginia B Andes Volunteer Community Clinic for a presentation to the Selby Foundation, which is considering our clinic for a grant. It's a significant amount of money and I hope we get it, but there is a lot of competition for a shrinking amount of available grant money these days. We put our best foot forward and I was proud to be able to report on all we have accomplished in the last year.

When I am not in doctor appointments I am working in the office or attending meetings, gatherings, dinners, fundraisers, and other outside activities. It seems like there is not enough time in the day to do everything. My routine these days is to start the day at 7 AM with a three-to-five mile walk or run with Moe (our dog) for 30 or 40 minutes. I never stop running once I am up and I am rarely home before 8 PM.

Tonight I came home to find out that doctors in Japan found a spot in the lung of my 52 year old Japanese bother-in-law. He's having a CT scan tomorrow. We'll know more by Friday. Let's pray this is not bad news.

Feeling Nostalgic for the Simple Life

When I was first diagnosed with lung cancer, I couldn't contemplate any future or make any plans. As time has gone on, however, things have returned to normal and I am again thinking about what comes next and what our life will be like down the road a bit. I am feeling so well these days, it is hard to imagine that I could relapse at any time.

Yoko and I are making travel plans for this summer. She has to return to Japan to attend her mother's seven year memorial service in August. It's customary in Japan to remember loved ones who have passed on the third and seventh anniversary of their death. So, Yoko and Jessie are going to Tokyo together at the end of July.

We decided that Yoko, Moe and I will drive to Blue Ridge, Georgia the week prior to her departure. We'll spend a few days together in a mountain cabin. Then, at the end of the week I will drive Yoko to Atlanta so she can catch a plane to Tokyo.

I'm going to return to Blue Ridge by myself while Yoko is gone and try to finish a screenplay I started years ago. A few weeks of uninterrupted effort is all I need to finally finish the job.

We decided to make a dry run and fly to Blue Ridge this weekend to check out cabins and become familiar with the place. When we return in the summer we'll take the car, but for this short weekend trip we decided to fly.

I have to say I am glad I don't travel by air as much as I once did. I can't stand the hassle and intrusion of airport security, the mobs of people, the delays and stress of making connections, the screaming babies who are invariably seated near you, and the airlines' consistently poor service. On this latest flight the "meal service" offered was a bag of salted peanuts. Yippee.

Lately I have become more acutely aware that our national life is changing and not for the better. Every day I wake up and things seem worse than they were before. Nothing is as it was and everything is more complex. Sometimes I wonder if simplifying and getting back to basics wouldn't be better.

In Blue Ridge today there was a "classic car" show on Main Street. Most of the cars being shown were beautifully restored models from the '50s and '60s. I could look at the gleaming, chrome-plated engines and actually see how everything fit together and worked. I can't say that if I look under the hood of a car today I could really tell what's what.

The log cabin we are staying in has all the modern conveniences, but none of the clutter. We have no neighbors and at night it is perfectly peaceful. We've been here only two days and I already feel like we've stayed a week. Living in a rustic setting has made me nostalgic for the past.

Tonight I made a fire on the cabin porch and shared a bottle of wine with Yoko as the sun was setting. I was recalling the days as a kid when we chased fireflies, toasted marshmallows on an open fire, and lay in the grass to watch the night sky for shooting stars. We had no worries and life was simple.

I don't often think about the past and what life was like when I was a child, but the uncertainty and complexity of the modern world has me yearning for those "good ole days".

Our trip to Blue Ridge this weekend happily coincided not only with Mother's Day, but Yoko and my 29th Wedding Anniversary and last night we watched a movie about divorce aptly called "It's Complicated." But really, it's simple. Stay married!

How to Maintain a Cancer Free Life

Ever since they suspended the clinical trial of the maintenance drug I was on, I have worried that I am doing nothing to proactively prevent a recurrence. I feel like I am just waiting around for cancer to strike again. It makes me uncomfortable and anxious. I would rather take the fight to the enemy than do nothing. So I have been reading up on things I can do on my own.

One of the best things I can do is fight this disease with nutrition. Everything that I have been reading has led me to believe that the key to cancer-free health is good nutrition. Fruits and vegetables that are high in antioxidants are known to be beneficial. I am drinking POM Wonderful (pomegranate juice) nearly every day.

I was approached by one multi-level marketer recently who recommended a drink called Xango, which is made from the mangosteen fruit. I tried a complementary bottle. It is better tasting than Mona Vie, which is made out of the acai berry, but I think they are in the same class of product — high priced juice drinks with potential (although unproven) health benefits. (I think I'd be just as well off with low-priced fruit juice concentrates from Publix.)

I've been complaining about our Food and Drug Administration for some weeks now because I don't see them doing anything useful, (except creating roadblocks and obstacles to cancer research and fretting about innocuous fruit drinks that may actually be helpful.)

As they did for POM Wonderful, the FDA did put out warning letters to the makers of both Xango and Mona Vie to not make medical claims about their products in their advertising. But does that mean these drinks don't have any medicinal benefit? No.

What I think it means is that they don't have any measured benefits meeting the FDA's scientific standards for a "drug."

This is the same FDA that recently approved the chemotherapy drug Tarceva (erlotinib) as maintenance therapy for patients with locally advanced metastatic lung cancer, despite a nearly unanimous (11-1) vote AGAINST expanded use of the drug by the FDA's own panel of experts who examined the evidence.

Why do you think the powers that be in the FDA overruled its own experts?

In the SATURN trial, nearly 900 patients with advanced non-small cell lung cancer received four cycles of first-line platinum-based chemotherapy. Patients were then split into two groups: one received placebo, and the other received maintenance Tarceva.

For patients on Tarceva, median progression-free survival (the time before the cancer progressed) reached 12.3 weeks, compared with 11.1 weeks for patients taking placebo. The Tarceva group lived only slightly longer, with median overall survival reaching 12 months for patients on Tarceva versus 11 months for those on placebo.

Sounds to me like Tarceva as a "maintenance drug" has as much benefit as POM Wonderful, Xango, or Mona Vie. Only Tarceva costs around $2,000 per month, about 20 times more than high-priced medicinal juice!

Until now Tarceva has been limited to use for advanced lung cancer that grew or spread after first line chemotherapy. Tarceva, an oral drug, is known to work well for those people who have the EGFR (epidermal growth factor receptor) gene mutation, which is only about 10% of lung cancer patients with non-small cell lung cancer.

At the National Lung Cancer Advocate Summit a few weeks ago, some of us fighting for lung cancer research were dumbfounded that the FDA would approve expanded use of Tarceva for maintenance therapy when we know that it does NOT work for most lung cancer patients.

OSI Pharmaceuticals, the maker of Tarceva, is surely pleased to now have approval to market their drug to a much larger universe of patients. It won't be long before we see TV commercials for the approved use, no doubt, urging lung cancer patients to "ask your doctor about Tarceva." It's an abomination.

Have We Lost the War on Cancer?

I watched a CBS "60 Minutes" story tonight about phthalates, a chemical that resides in nearly everything made of plastic that needs to be soft and flexible — shower curtains, beach balls, rubber ducks, to name but a few. These chemicals, which are used in thousands of everyday items, are allegedly linked to deformity in male genitalia, congenital hernias and changes in the hormonal balances of men. But is it really any surprise that chemicals (of any sort) in our environment have a potential negative impact on our health or our progeny?

The experts that accuse phthalates of having potential to do harm cannot say anything definitive about the toxic effect of these chemicals without "more data". And, of course, the chemical manufacturers that make these substances deny there is any linkage to birth deformities, even though data proving this does not exist. Last year congress, "split the baby", so to speak, by banning certain phthalates from use in toys.

When I was a kid, it seemed like we were a nation that had all the answers. John Wayne and the Lone Ranger persuaded me that the good guys in white hats always prevailed. Right won over might, usually just in the nick of time.

I grew up in an America that gloried in winning World War II. When I was a kid our nation was fighting communism and the Cold War. We were the predominant economic power having invented and manufactured many of the world's modern conveniences — the electric light, the automobile, the telephone, the airplane, the transistor, and the television. I was seven years old when John Kennedy inspired our nation to reach for the stars. In less than 10 years we landed on the moon. It seemed there was nothing we couldn't do.

In my lifetime, America has always been the leading political, military, economic and technological power. It still is, but I have to say that, lately, my faith in America to get to the truth, figure out what's right for the nation, and move forward with good public policy has been shaken.

I have a hard time fathoming that we could allow drilling in the ocean with deep water rigs and not have a contingency plan for a blow-out oil disaster, like the one unfolding in the Gulf. Are you kidding me? Isn't it common sense that the government would require contingency disaster plans before issuing permits for offshore drilling? All I can say is that if they didn't imagine this kind of thing could happen, they don't have much of an imagination, which brings me to the topic of government sponsored cancer research.

Richard Nixon declared a "War on Cancer" in 1971, yet here we are nearly four decades later no closer to a cure than we were back then. In fact, no one talks about a cure any longer. Today, we only speak of treatments.

The basic approach to treating cancer has not changed in 50 years. The tools are new and improved, but the strategy is the same — search and destroy cancerous cells using chemotherapy, surgery and radiation. There is nothing new or radically innovative or imaginative in our approach, so it's hard to see how the outcome will change. As my father use to say, doing the same thing over and over and expecting a different result is the definition of insanity. Perhaps it's finally time to look at other approaches.

Someone recommended that I read Suzanne Somers's book "Knockout: Interviews with Doctors Who Are Curing Cancer." I purchased a copy to see what she had to say. The doctors she interviewed have interesting new strategies about curing cancer that does not involve search and destroy treatments. Why aren't some of these non-toxic "cures" being seriously tested? First I need to find an oncologist even willing to read the book.

Getting the Incentives Right

I never took psychology in school and it is definitely one of my weak points. I am not good at using psychology, because I am ignorant of even its very basic tenets. I read a book called "On Success" by famed investor Charlie Munger, who talked about how important psychology is in business and management. After reading what he had to say, I really felt like there was a huge hole in my education.

Munger, who was self-taught in psychology, came up with his own list of human tendencies or behavioral patterns, one of which he calls the "Reward and Punishment Super Response Tendency." This is the first on his list of twenty-five human tendencies, in recognition of how important incentive and disincentive is to human behavior. Munger summarizes the issue with a famous quote from a Soviet worker: "They pretend to pay us and we pretend to work." Munger says that the most important rule in management is to "get the incentives right."

He describes how Federal Express at first struggled to get packages shifted rapidly between aircraft at the central hub each night. Everything they tried did not get the task accomplished quickly enough. Then someone had the brilliant idea to pay the night shift by the shift, rather than by the hour, and let them go home early if all the planes were loaded. That simple and elegant solution worked.

Munger talks about what he calls "incentive-caused bias" that leads to immoral behavior. His example is a surgeon in Lincoln Nebraska who removed "bushel baskets full of normal healthy gallbladders". This medical fraud was rationalized by the surgeon, who believed the gallbladder was the source of all disease. He was well paid to exercise his talent, whether the patient needed the gallbladder removed or not. HE was eventually removed from the medical profession and rightly charged with malpractice.

Incentive-caused bias is prevalent in every business and profession. Bad or immoral behavior, according to Munger, is "intensely habit forming when well rewarded." We have certainly seen many examples of this in recent years. Enron's manipulative accounting misdeeds, Bernie Madoff's gigantic Ponzi scheme, the whole residential mortgage debacle, are examples of immoral behavior well rewarded. In my profession, it's the insurance salesman whose only and every answer to making an investment recommendation is an annuity that pays a high commission.

It appears to me that poorly designed incentives and controls are at the core of bad behavior in every case.

There's an old saying that," if the only tool in the drawer is a hammer, every problem looks like a nail." We keep banging away at cancer, using chemo, radiation and surgery without getting significantly better results. Could it be that alternative treatments are less lucrative than the orthodox treatments and therefore not pursued? Are cancer patients the unwitting victims of incentive-caused bias by the medical profession?

Munger muses that the cash register was a great moral instrument when it was created. It ended the inventor's employees from stealing him blind. Widespread incentive-caused bias in all human endeavors causes Munger to distrust professional advice, especially if it is good for the advisor. How would Munger feel if he were a cancer patient?

I got to thinking about this incentive-caused bias in relation to cancer treatment. It makes me wonder if drug companies, insurance companies and the medical industry as a whole, are properly incentivized to do what is best for patients. Certainly that should be the goal, but incentive-caused bias may make some treatment alternatives more attractive than others.

What is the equivalent of the cash register when it comes to treating cancer? The role of government regulation should be to ensure that the medical industry does what is best for patients. Maybe we should start by examining the incentive-caused bias in medicine. Reform needs to ensure that we get the incentives right.

Back in the Saddle

When my children were little, we lived in Tokyo, where I worked for the now defunct accounting firm, Arthur Andersen & Co. Yoko's parents only lived 30 minutes away and we would regularly go to visit.

Japanese homes are very small and not conducive to having company, so it wouldn't be long before someone would suggest that we take the kids to the park. Yoko's parents lived across the street from "*Baji Koen*" – literally translated "Equestrian Park" where our girls played on the swings and jungle gyms. From time to time there would be horse shows taking place at the park, which was built as the equestrian venue for the 1964 Olympics.

After admiring the skill of the riders in a show one year, I casually remarked to Yoko that it would be fun to learn to ride. Yoko took me seriously and within a week or two made it happen. After doing some investigation, she discovered the riding school Avalon, less than five minutes from our home.

We would go to Avalon on the weekends to hang out in the coffee shop and watch the riders practicing in the arena for hours on end. Eventually I enrolled in the school, bought the necessary riding equipment, and began to learn the skills of dressage and show-jumping.

Like any sport or activity in Japan, equestrian riding has a ranking system. You have to show proficiency at each level to advance to the next. After about five years of riding I became a top ranked rider, licensed to show in competition. At some point along the way I needed to have my own horse in order to advance. That lead to the purchase of an Arabian we named Tis Adore. For about five years my life outside of work was largely spent at Avalon riding and grooming horses.

Once I left the employ of Arthur Andersen, it was hard to keep up with the expense of stabling a horse in Tokyo. Sadly, I had to give up Tis Adore and riding in 1995. I have not been on a horse since until recently.

People who don't ride generally don't realize what an extremely aerobic sport it is. While it may look as though the horse is doing all the work, the rider is using nearly every muscle in his or her body to maintain proper "seat" and balance and keep the horse relaxed and under control. I remember the first time I jumped a horse in a show; I rode a fairly easy circuit in about one minute. I was astonished to find that my legs were so weakened that I could hardly stand after dismounting.

I have not been on a strenuous exercise regimen since I gave up riding. I golf every week, ride a bike or walk the dog every day, but none of these produces the aerobic exercise I know I need. Joining a gym to run or lifting weights is just not my thing. I would rather play a sport or do something that produces a sweat.

A friend of mine has been caring for two horses here at a local stables. Her daughter rides. The second horse has issues and is not being exercised much. Knowing that I use to ride, I was invited down to see the horse and take her around the arena. It's been nearly 15 years since I have been on a horse. I was happy to know that after all these years I could still remember the basics.

Good Process/Good Results

I have to say I have become very cynical about the world. Maybe it's because I am getting older and have gained some perspective. Or was I naïve for most of my life? I never considered people's motives when it came to healthcare, science, the law, economic policy, and the like.

I am realizing how devoted people are to their own self-interest, which, I have to say, it is disheartening. I grew up when "Camelot" was all the rage on Broadway. I thought people, in general, were "pure of heart" and self-sacrificing, like Lancelot. I wish the world were so.

I had a discussion this week with a fellow at the office about the financial regulatory reform measures now winding their way through Congress. I don't know what the end result will be, but I do suspect that there is more than politics as usual going on. My friend's thesis is that the Democrats are driving the process in such a way as to be in a position to squeeze Wall Street for greater campaign contributions for the upcoming fall elections in exchange for less onerous regulation. Is this really the way the system should work? Are politicians gaming legislative processes as a way of squeezing campaign contributions from Wall Street?

President Obama has said that he would use "every resource at his disposal" to deal with the oil spill in the Gulf, yet he has refused to accept offers of aid from 13 countries. Some countries have superior technology to fight an offshore spill of this magnitude. According to one story I read, Dutch and Belgian dredgers have the technology in-house and special vessels to fight the spill, but the Jones Act, protectionist legislation passed in the 1920's, prevents them from working in the US. The Jones Act requires that all goods transported by water between U.S. ports be carried in U.S.-flag ships, constructed in the United States, owned by U.S. citizens, and crewed by U.S. citizens and U.S. permanent residents.

In a national emergency Obama could waive the requirements of the Jones Act, but he has failed to act. In the face of this disaster you have to wonder why? Could it be that he doesn't want to offend his labor union supporters?

I'm a big believer in "good process, good results." In fact, it is how the Japanese learned to manufacture quality goods. W. Edwards Deming, an American statistician, taught the Japanese statistical techniques used to dissect processes to learn what leads to bad results. The goal was to improve the process and thereby improve the results. Today the Japanese strive for perfection and zero defects. We Americans seem to be satisfied with standards that are "within tolerance." Another way to say it is tolerable (not necessarily good) results.

Good processes do not always result in good outcomes, but it certainly improves the chances of getting things right. We need to be constantly asking ourselves if the processes we have in place are going to help us get the results we are looking for. Speaking of which…

I went for my CT/Pet Scan this week and was anxious to hear the results, so I sat with the radiologist after the scans were completed and we reviewed the pictures together, from head to toe. Thankfully, the radiologist could find no evidence of disease. It is the best of all possible outcomes and I am so grateful to be alive and healthy. I am now looking forward to marking my third anniversary of life since my diagnosis.

Thinking about this makes me wonder if it was just luck or something else that has kept me alive to date. I think good process has been integral to my recovery. We had a plan. We worked the plan systematically. We used all available resources to get the best possible outcome, and it worked!

Let's pray the Gulf of Mexico is as lucky.

Research Breakthroughs and the Road Ahead

On Friday I got a phone call from the clinic that is conducting the clinical trial for Stimuvax, the trial drug I am taking. The research had been suspended because patients in the trial, for unknown reasons, had developed encephalitis. The phone call was to let me know that the trial had now been given the green light to go forward. I am due to get my next shots tomorrow.

Every six weeks for the past two years I have travelled to New Port Richey to receive these vaccinations. I will continue to go for the shots until there is progression of the disease, which is the first endpoint of the study. In the Phase II trials of this drug, time to progression was 36 months for people on Stimuvax versus 17 months for those taking a placebo. In August I will have been on the drug for 24 months. While I don't know if I am getting the drug or a placebo, I've always suspected I was getting the drug. My continued good health is nothing short of a miracle.

The theory of Stimuvax is that it works to boost your immune system to fight cancerous cells — not exactly a novel idea. This was the approach used by Dr. Royal Rife back in the 1930s; it is also the approach being used by various alternative treatment practitioners highlighted in Suzanne Somers' book, "Knockout." Interestingly, strengthening the body's immune system to fight cancer is now becoming more of the conventional wisdom in drug therapy. At the ASCO (American Society of Clinical Oncology) Convention in Chicago last month study results from several new drugs that target the immune system got a lot of attention in the press.

One drug, ipilimumab, from Bristol Myers, is designed to enhance the immune system and increase the survival rate for people with advanced melanoma, a deadly form of skin cancer. Patients taking the new drug lived an average of 10 months versus six months for patients taking a comparison drug, GP100. More than 45% of patients taking the new drug were alive after one year, compared with 25% of the patients who received the GP100 vaccine. Ipilimumab is a monoclonal antibody, a biologic drug derived from living cells. It works by activating T-cells, part of the immune system, to help fight cancer cell growth.

Targeting drugs for people with certain genetic mutations also seems to be the wave of the future. Pfizer is now testing the drug crizotinib, which appears to shrink tumors in lung cancer patients with certain genetic mutations. The discovery was a lucky happenstance. Pfizer initially thought crizotinib would work to inhibit C-met, an enzyme that is alleged to feed tumor growth. Company researchers noticed that the drug also worked on another enzyme, anaplastic lymphoma kinase or ALK, also thought to be involved with tumor growth. Researchers in Japan subsequently found that fusion of ALK with another gene was a contributor to lung cancer. Roughly 3-5% of lung cancer patients or about 40,000 people annually worldwide, have the ALK mutation.

Pfizer conducted a clinical trial on patients who have the mutation. Most were either light smokers or never smoked. The average age was 50. The drug, an oral pill, was taken twice daily. Results so far are very promising. Of the 82 patients tested, roughly 90% experienced tumor shrinkage or stabilization. Pfizer is now moving on to the Stage III Clinic trial.

The ASCO Convention also saw the announcement of two new drugs — Sprycel and Tasigna, to treat leukemia and possibly replace the miracle drug, Gleevec, which has been the standard of care for leukemia since it was first introduced in 2001.

I'm happy that research is finally starting to get somewhere. It is heartening to know that new avenues of treatment may be available to me down the road.

The National Lung Cancer Partnership Annual Summit

I've just returned from the annual three-day lung cancer advocate summit, organized by the National Lung Cancer Partnership. I don't know where to begin. All I can say is WOW; I wish you could have been there.

I went to the summit last year in Dallas. This year the event was held in Tampa, with the support of The H. Lee Moffitt Cancer Center. There were 108 advocates in attendance. Twenty four were lung cancer survivors. Many others were there to honor the memory of a father, mother, sister, brother or friend who lost their battle with lung cancer.

On the first night there was a cocktail reception and dinner. I saw a lot of my friends from last year's conference and met a host of newcomers. During dinner everyone in attendance was asked to introduce themselves and say where they were from and why they had come. To say the least, emotions ran very high in the room as story after story was shared about how this disease not only unfairly took the life of a loved one, but devastated the people they left behind.

It was a very moving and powerful way to start the conference. You would have to have a heart of stone not to be choked with emotion as you listened to all the reasons people want to become involved and advocate for lung cancer awareness, research and change.

For example, at my table was a young woman named Emily, who is 34 years old. Emily was recently diagnosed with Stage IV lung cancer. She never smoked a day in her life (yet the first thing people ask when they learn she has lung cancer is, "Did you smoke?") She is the young mother of a daughter who just turned three.

Emily believes that estrogen during pregnancy may have had something to do with the rapid growth of her tumor and the resulting terminal diagnosis. Researchers suspect estrogen may play some role in the development of lung cancer as it does with breast cancer, but again, more research is needed. Emily wants answers about why many young mothers are developing lung cancer. She wants to advocate for research on the causes of lung cancer in women and non-smokers.

Another mother I had a chance to speak with was there for her 22-year-old son, who just had returned from serving in Iraq. He was home for only a few months and was about to be discharged from the service when his Stage IV cancer was diagnosed. He only survived for a few months after his diagnosis, leaving behind his wife and newborn son. That mother wants answers too.

And then there were two young sisters — Stephanie Weis and Jennifer Melton — who were getting involved because their father had recently lost his battle with lung cancer at the age of 59. They wrote a beautifully illustrated children's book called "Pink Sky at Night" in honor of their father. There was not a dry eye in the house as the girls sobbed relating the love they had for their father and the hole his death has left in their hearts. Proceeds from the sale of their book will go to lung cancer research.

US Cancer Deaths vs. Federal Research Funding per Death

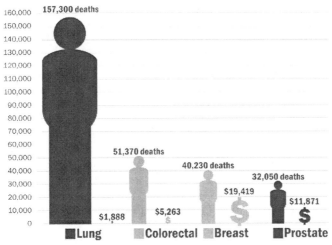

Figure ©2011 National Lung Cancer Partnership. All rights reserved.

Estimated deaths by cancer type in the U.S. for 2010 are from the American Cancer Society Facts and Figures, 2010: http://www.cancer.org/Research/CancerFactsFigures/CancerFactsFigures/cancer-facts-and-figures-2010

Annual funding figures represent the National Cancer Institute (NCI) and Department of Defense estimated 2010 spending*:
NCI: http://budgettool.cancer.gov/budget-spending/funding-by-cancer-type/fiscal-year-2010.aspx
Department of Defense Lung, Breast, and Prostate Research Program descriptions available at http://cdmrp.army.mil/researchprograms.shtml
*While the Centers for Disease Control & Prevention (CDC) also funds cancer research, a breakdown of spending between research and public health interventions is not currently available.

Lung cancer is the number one cause of cancer deaths, accounting for more deaths than breast, prostate and colon cancer combined. Twice as many women will die from lung cancer than from breast cancer, yet lung cancer only receives a small fraction of the available cancer funding. Why?

Leaving the summit last year motivated me to organize the first Free to Breathe 5K Run/Walk event held in Florida to raise money for lung cancer research. My motivation now is even higher.

We Are Who We Came From

Everyone has a story and everyone's story is complex. You can't boil down someone's life or who they are into just a few words.

My life started when I was born to my father and mother. They, in turn, were the product of their parents.

My grandfather on my father's side was from Melfi Potenza in southern Italy, near Naples. I know he worked as a barber, but other than that I don't remember anything about my grandfather. I was very young when he died. He was only in his 60s. What I know about my grandfather comes from the stories my father told about him. I know he had a temper and was strict. I also know he had a sense of humor and liked to sneak around the house scaring my grandmother by jumping out of closets.

My paternal grandmother was an Italian born in Tunisia. Her father was a commercial trader working in North Africa when Tunisia was an Italian colony. My grandmother was famous for being emotional. She would cry at our every coming and going. She was a great cook. Whenever I think of her I think of the fresh Italian bread she would bake for us.

My grandparents were both immigrants who were processed through Ellis Island in the early 20th century.

My mother was the oldest daughter of Timothy and Mary (Moody) Donovan — pure Irish. Both my grandfathers were doughboys in World War I and fought in France under General Pershing. My grandfather on my mother's side worked as a road construction supervisor for the City of Bristol. I grew up knowing both of my maternal grandparents, who died in their late 90s.

I have a family tree on mother's side that traces the Moody lineage back to 1821. Unfortunately, all we have are names, dates of birth and dates of death. There are few stories associated with any of these names.

There are great stories about all the people who came before me. Yoko has her own family history in Japan. Our children are the beneficiaries of all their Japanese, Italian and Irish roots. It's a shame that we don't know more to pass on to future generations.

The Japanese have a tradition of remembering their ancestors. In fact, this week Yoko and daughter Jessica are returning to Japan to commemorate the 7th anniversary of Yoko's mother's passing. Yoko remembers her parents and my father every day by placing a small offering of tea before their pictures and saying a silent prayer to ask for their blessings.

Her prayers were answered this week with news that my daughter, Paula, and Brian are having a baby. We're delighted about now becoming grandparents ourselves! Now I hope I'll have the chance to be a grandfather to remember. There is so much I want to pass on!

My First Staycation

One of my life's ambitions has been to write something that would be published as a book or made into a movie. Since being diagnosed with cancer, I've realized how quickly time passes. I feel an urgent need to realize this ambition, so I am taking two weeks to work on my writing projects at home. It's the first time I have had a "staycation."

Since Yoko and I have been married, we have taken numerous family trips and vacations. Most of the time, we were so busy on vacation we would arrive back home more exhausted than when we left!

When I worked in Japan for Arthur Andersen, we were allowed two weeks for home leave, all expenses paid. Typically we would fly home from Japan using a direct flight, but sometimes we would plan our trip to spend time in Hawaii, one of my favorite vacation destinations. Stopping in Hawaii was a great way to transition between time zones and cultures and get a little caught up on sleep.

Home leave trips usually entailed a combination of vacation time with obligatory family visits, since we rarely had the chance to get home to see everyone. Between the time required for travel and visiting relatives, there was rarely little time left for real rest and relaxation.

When we lived in San Francisco for a brief period in the 80s, we were busy just trying to get established. Money was tight and time was scarce. I remember taking Yoko and Paula, who was a baby, to Trinity Lake in the Cascades for a long weekend in June one year. The scenery was peaceful and beautiful. The mountains were still snowcapped and we were in the middle of a gigantic lake in a huge national forest. No one was around. Yoko, who was born and raised in the big city, was scared that we would be attacked by animals, mugged by drifters, or be stranded without help in some remote cove. It was a nice vacation idea but, between bears, raccoons scratching around and the bats at night, it turned out to be less than restful.

One of my favorite vacations spots on the planet is Jackson Hole, Wyoming. In fact, we liked it so much the first time we went, we ended up buying a vacation rental on a butte overlooking the Grand Tetons. I remember one year going with Yoko and the kids to ski for Christmas. With the highest vertical drop in North America and light powdered snow, Jackson Hole is a fantastic place to ski, but what a hassle to get there and then return with ski equipment, winter clothing, gifts, etc.! Sadly, we went only once for a winter wonderland vacation.

Because getting out of Japan was so expensive and time consuming, we took short weekend vacations. We sometimes took the kids to Club Med in Hokkaido. You could fly to Sahoro from nearby Haneda Airport in about one hour and be on the ski slopes by late afternoon. While the kids were being entertained, Yoko and I could go off to enjoy ourselves without worry.

I had always wanted to take our family to Europe on vacation but never had the chance, because it was so far from Japan. After Hurricane Charley destroyed our house in August of 2004, I decided to take all the girls to London and Paris for a week, just to get out of town and give everyone something good to remember for that year. By that time, however, Paula was working and couldn't go.

Yoko and Jessie left today for Japan for a two-week visit to see family and friends. I am at home with the dog reading, writing, and enjoying my first "staycation". No cost. No jetlag. No bags. Yeah baby! Now that's what I call a vacation!

The Clinical Trial Bottleneck

I always thought that clinical trials were something you considered doing as a patient when there were no other treatment options available. It made sense to me that you would try all the conventional treatment options first and then, if all else failed, resort to trial drugs. It's a fair assumption, but it's wrong. In many cases, using a trial drug first may be the better option.

A newly diagnosed cancer patient may not typically think to ask their physician what trials are available to them before beginning "standard of care" treatments. Most physicians themselves are not familiar with all of the trials available and the eligibility criteria for participation. A quick search for lung cancer trials currently recruiting patients at the National Institutes of Health's website (www.clincialtrial.gov) reveals that there are more than 1,000 open trials related to cancer alone. There is no way to easily find a trial other than to do a search and narrow down or refine the criteria to meets your needs, condition and location. In many cases it will be up to the patient to find a clinical trial and then consult with their physician about the benefits of participating.

Clinical trials are an important part of cancer research and medical research in general. Unfortunately, the "accrual rates" for many studies are so low that trials are frequently closed for lack of participation. It's estimated that only 3% of newly diagnosed cancer patients enroll in clinical trials — an exceedingly low number. I saw one study on this topic that declared that more than 40% of all oncology trials "don't meet the minimum target for patient accruals."

Clinical trials are the bottleneck to faster advancement in cancer research. We all have a stake in seeing cancer research advance more rapidly. A recent report from the National Cancer Institute estimates that 41 percent of Americans living today will develop cancer in their lifetime; one in four will eventually die from the disease.

One study that looked into the reasons for low accrual rates for cancer patients in clinical trials reveals that of the 276 patients studied only 14 percent ultimately participated in a trial. The most common reasons for patients not participating were elimination by their physician because of perceived availability or poor performance status; the desire for other treatment and distance from the available trial sites.

The Phase III Stimuvax trial I am enrolled in requires 1,200 patients be recruited. There are 259 sites around the world participating in this particular trial with four here in Florida. It may take five years or more before 1,200 patients are accrued and the study completed.

Before joining a trial, a participant must qualify for the study. Some research studies seek participants with illnesses or conditions to be studied, while others need healthy participants. Clinical trials require that patient sign a document that explains the risks and benefits of the trial, called an informed consent.

American Food Culture

I have never been heavy, but since I was diagnosed with cancer, I have put on a few pounds. Actually, I've gained more than a few. I am 5 foot 10 inches tall and for most of my adult life, while living in Japan, I weighed less than 140 pounds. That's pretty skinny.

I started gaining weight when we moved back from Japan in 1998. When I was diagnosed with cancer in 2007 I weighed about 150 pounds. During chemo and radiation treatment I lost a few pounds but since then I have continually gained weight. As of this writing I weigh 165 pounds and rising.

So why am I gaining weight? Well, one reason is my metabolism has slowed. It used to be that I could eat like a horse, drink like a fish, and not gain an ounce. Lately I have to watch what I eat and drink.

The main reason for my weight gain is what I put in my mouth. We eat and drink a lot of sweet things in this country and, as Yoko will tell you, I love sweet things, like pies, cookies, ice cream, and candy. When I lived in Japan I did not consume as much sweets as I do here. At work in Japan we would drink unsweetened hot green tea. Here I drink coffee with sugar and cream throughout the day. There is no question that hot green tea is better for you and less fattening.

A third reason for my weight gain has to do with the amount of exercise I get. I get in my car and drive to and from work. In fact, I drive everywhere. I'm walking the dog or riding my bike in the morning before work as a way to purposely get some exercise, but, obviously it is not enough. Fattening foods and the convenience of living a lazy middle-class American lifestyle lends itself to weight gain.

In contrast, my daily routine in Japan was embedded with good eating and exercise. I typically walked 15 minutes to the train station in the morning and home again in the evening. During the day I would walk to and from the subway station and up and down stairs and then walk to appointments. I easily walked two or three miles a day as well as up and down 10 to 15 stories of stairs. In short, I lead a pretty healthy lifestyle that allowed me to stay trim.

Of course, I ate a lot of fish and rice in Japan as well as steamed vegetables. The Japanese don't use much butter or oil in their cooking and bread is not served with a Japanese meal. The only really bad thing the Japanese use regularly as an ingredient is soy sauce, which is high in sodium. Generally the Japanese don't fry a lot of food in oil or eat a lot of meat. They boil things in water, steam-cook foods, grill, or prepare foods raw (like sushi or sashimi). Japanese cuisine is often described as "delicate." Some might say "bland." Meals are generally light and prepared in numerous small dishes. Steamed white rice is the staple. Japanese food culture offers a wide variety in tastes and textures.

Both Yoko and I bemoan America's food culture and our unhealthy eating habits. We both think Americans generally lack education about good food and healthy eating. We find it hard to believe, for example, that children are allowed to choose what they eat at school. Do we really expect kids to make healthy food choices? It is little wonder that there is a growing obesity crisis in this country.

School lunch in Japan is determined by a committee of parents who collectively decide on what their kids eat each day. Maybe that's where we should start to change our food culture.

Managing Cancer Care and Diabetes

I was very lucky. When I was diagnosed with lung cancer nearly three years ago I was symptomatic (I had a persistent cough) but thankfully I did not have any complicating issues or disease.

I did not know at the time that the medical world uses a scoring system to quantify a patient's general well-being. I had a "performance status" of one when I was diagnosed (symptomatic but completely ambulatory.). A performance status indicating generally good health allowed my doctors to treat me without needing to account for how treatments would affect some other disease. Today I would be scored a zero (asymptomatic, fully active and able to carry on all activities without restriction.) If I have a cancer recurrence, my general good health should help me fight the disease. These days I work hard at trying to stay healthy.

I say I was lucky, because people with cancer frequently have other medical issues, such as diabetes, high blood pressure, kidney disease, COPD, and so on. These patients are understandably more challenging for an oncologist to treat effectively.

I was surprised to learn that diabetics, despite seeing a doctor more often than most other people, appear to be less likely to be screened for cancer. That is disturbing on a number of fronts, not the least of which is the suspicion that there exists some link between cancer and diabetes. In fact, one estimate I found is that cancer rates among diabetics may be as high as 18%. The link between these two diseases is as yet unproven. Nevertheless, you would think that, given the high rate of cancer among diabetics, screening rates would be higher, not lower.

One Canadian study showed that the mammography rates for women with diabetes were more than 30% below their nondiabetic counterparts. The low screening rates in that study were attributed to "time constraints during office visits for complex disease care." The upshot is that if you are diabetic, you may want to ask your physician about cancer screening and prevention.

Diabetic patients present treatment challenges for oncologists. For example, many diabetic patients may have pre-existing issues with their kidney or heart or suffer from neuropathy. All of theses conditions may be exacerbated by chemotherapy, depending on the agent being used. Cisplatin, which is what I was given, is known to impair the kidneys and cause peripheral neuropathy. But successful treatment typically requires that 85% of the chemo-therapeutic dose be given. Reducing the treatment dosage or timing to temper side effects may also affect the treatment's efficacy. It is a difficult choice to have to make.

Diabetics face other challenges in being treated for cancer, with the largest being control of blood sugar levels. Treatment induced nausea and vomiting, for example, can be controlled with drugs, but steroid based anti-nausea drugs may, in turn, wreak havoc on controlling blood sugar levels and the amount of insulin a patient is required to take. Being able to maintain proper nutrition during cancer treatment is a challenge for a diabetic.

While the link between diabetes and cancer is not yet definitive, there are many common risk factors, including age, obesity, poor diet and lack of exercise. Prevention of diabetes is an important factor in fighting all cancers. People with diabetes double the risk of developing liver and pancreatic cancer. It is known to increase the risk for colorectal, breast and bladder cancer by 20% to 50%. In contrast, for some unknown reason, prostate cancer is less prevalent in men with diabetes. Go figure.

Research presented at ASCO this year showed that metformin, a drug commonly used in the treatment of type-2 diabetes, helped guard against tobacco-induced lung cancer in mice. More research is needed to see if this commonly used drug to treat diabetes is a potential lung cancer preventative in humans. Let's hope research progresses soon.

Fooled By Randomness

Nassim Nicholas Taleb has written another best seller called "Fooled by Randomness — The Hidden Role of Chance in Life and in the Markets."

I think everyone should read this book because it provides great perspective about life in general. I've been reading the book as a way of getting a handle on risk management in the current economic climate, but I am finding that the concepts Taleb explains could be applied to all facets of life. If you can get past the author's obvious intellectual snobbery, it's a pretty good read.

If I had to sum up his concepts, it's the idea that we human beings are blind to the role that probability and randomness (luck, both good and bad) plays in our daily lives. We tend to take credit for our hard work and skill, if we succeed in life, and we often blame ourselves if we fail. But we didn't choose where we were born or our parents or the time period in which we live. I'm glad I was not born in Haiti. I'm glad my mother cared for me and was not a crack addict. I've been lucky.

Taleb says we commonly mistake luck for skill. He illustrates this concept in numerous ways. One example that illustrates alternative outcomes goes like this. Imagine I provide you with a loaded revolver and offer to pay you $10 million each time you put the gun to your head and pull the trigger. The revolver has six chambers but only one holds a bullet. Before the game begins, there are five potentially happy outcomes and one fatal result. If you live, it doesn't mean you're skilled, it means you are lucky and brave, even though the odds are with you that you'll survive!

Imagine a money manager that has five market beating years in a row. We infer from the manager's track record that he is skilled, when in fact it may just be luck to have been in the right asset class or using a strategy that works in most circumstances. You might hire him because of his good track record, mistaking luck for skill. Past performance is not indicative of future results!

You can apply that concept to nearly any human endeavor. For example, like tens of thousands of other people, I am working on writing a screenplay. Most screenplays started will never be finished, even fewer will ever be read by the right people and only a handful of the plays that are read will be made into a movie. Writing a successful movie script has as much to do with luck as it does with the skill of the writer.

One thing I can say for sure is that if I don't write the screenplay, I can never be a screenplay writer. (If I don't pull the trigger, I can never win the $10 million.) It comes down to what you are willing to risk. As Clint Eastwood would say, "Do you feel lucky?"

In the last few weeks I have had numerous conversations with people of all walks of life who are struggling in the current economy. I think people feel that they have done something wrong or made the wrong choices. Somehow they feel they are to blame for loss of a job, income or wealth. Nothing could be further from the truth. It's just bad luck and it's not over till the fat lady sings. Better days are ahead.

I've gone through good times and bad times in my life. The ups and downs of living are part of the randomness of events we don't easily see and can't predict.

Einstein railed against the idea of random chance in physics. He is known for the famous quote that "God does not play dice." I don't agree. God invented the game and enjoys watching how we react to our daily wins and losses.

The Law is a Poor Substitute for Morality

It is too bad that we think that the law can be a substitute for common sense, decency or fair play. It can't be. We Americans are all about protecting our rights under the law and our freedoms. But don't we also have a moral obligation to do what is right for society at large? Isn't the price for freedom about doing the right thing without having to create a law in the first place?

If everyone just did what was plainly right and commonly seen as being in the public interest, there would be less need for laws and lawyers. We have 1.1 million lawyers in the United States. Japan, which has a population half our size, has just 23,000 active attorneys. How does Japan get along with so few attorneys?

Here in America, anything that is not explicitly outlawed is deemed to be "legal." It is just the opposite in Japan. If it is not explicitly allowed by the law, you should assume it is illegal. The Japanese system provides regulators with wide discretionary authority to decide what is allowed and what is not.

I am frustrated and angry with how people follow "the letter of the law," but pervert and abuse the clear intent of the law. Take the ban on marketing cigarettes to children. When I attended a Tobacco-Free Charlotte County meeting organized by the

Charlotte County Health Department last week, I learned for the first time how tobacco companies are getting around the prohibition of marketing cigarettes to minors. It really makes me mad.

For example, I didn't know that you could convert cigarettes into "cigars" to get around the law, simply by changing the packaging. I had never heard of nicotine laced toothpicks, swizzle sticks, lip-balm, candy flavored tobacco (snuff) and candy-flavored nicotine drops that look like harmless breath mints.

To me nicotine laced products are all drug delivery systems that should simply be banned. Now that the FDA has the authority to regulate the manufacturing, marketing and sale of tobacco products, I hope they'll get to work. In the meantime, tobacco companies and others continue to devise new ways to evade the law and create a new generation of addicts. It is reprehensible.

There is hardly a person in this country who doesn't know that nicotine is a habit forming, potentially lethal substance. Nicotine laced products, including smokeless tobacco, are being marketed under the guise of being smoking-cessation products. In reality many of these products are being used as just another way of turning our kids into nicotine addicts. Who do they think they are kidding?

What's the harm of nicotine-laced products? It is widely assumed that tar and other substances in tobacco smoke are the cancer causing agents in cigarettes. Get rid of the smoke and you get rid of the problem. But recent studies have made a strong connection between nicotine itself and cancer. The thought is that, over time, nicotine impairs the immune system and your body's ability to fight and destroy cancer cells.

To avoid the high federal excise tax on cigarettes, tobacco retailers are now taking advantage of a loophole in the law with new "roll your own" machines. The new machines, being deployed at tobacco shops across the country, produce a carton of cigarettes in about eight minutes using loose tobacco, which is exempt from federal taxes. A carton of roll your own costs just $21, about half the price of a carton of regular cigarettes.

When an existing law does not do what it was intended to do, we enact more laws to close such "loopholes." The fact is that people who are intent on circumventing the law will always find a work around. If it is very profitable and illegal they'll just go underground. The law is surely no substitute for morality.

The Role of Faith in Healing

This week there was a news story about how the famed British physicist, Stephen Hawking, concluded that the laws of physics are such that God is not necessary for the universe to have been formed. Spontaneous creation is possible, he says, without the intervention of a divine being. I say, fair enough, but then, how have the physical laws of the universe come about? If the universe "just exists" in infinite time, does life's struggles have no meaning? I find that hard to believe. As a victim of ALS, Hawking must surely have doubts too.

For thirty years my wife and I have discussed and argued over the topic of God and religion. I'm not sure we have ever fully agreed on anything, except that everyone should be free to believe whatever their hearts tell them to believe. When it came to religion we struggled with what we should teach our children. For example, if, as taught by Christianity, no one can enter the kingdom of heaven except through our Lord Savior, Jesus Christ, does that mean Yoko's loving parents (who were faithful Buddhists) are to be left outside the pearly gates for all eternity? Neither Yoko nor I believe God would be so arbitrary or cruel.

Yoko and I agree that no one can claim to have a definitive answer when it comes to the hereafter, if there is such a thing. So why argue over it? What you believe is a matter of faith — whether you are an atheist, Buddhist, Hindi, Christian, Muslim or Jew. Ultimately we concluded that our children should think for themselves and discover on their own what it is they believe.

I believe that faith comes from within and is held within our heart. True faith can't be taught or learned. It is something we feel and know intuitively. It is literally our sixth sense.

I believe faith and spirituality has a real physical effect on our health and well-being. Invariably when people are sick or feeling hopeless, they turn to God. "We'll keep you in our prayers" is the refrain of the faithful.

From my experience people with deep religious faith exhibit a certain calm and acceptance when faced with the diagnosis of a devastating disease. Faith may actually help them to recover. Studies have shown that people who attend church regularly are less likely to suffer from hypertension, exhibit lower death rates after certain kinds of surgery, and recover more quickly from serious illness.

The explanation is not necessarily attributable to an intervening God. People who attend church regularly have more social support than non-churchgoers, generally have healthier lifestyles, and are better able to cope with stress, which weakens the immune system. Simply believing that God heals (whether God plays an active role or not) may contribute to the healing process.

We become more serious about God when we're sick because a serious illness forces us to consider our mortality. We have a sudden realization that death eventually comes to all of us. We want to believe that life has meaning and our "end" marks the beginning of our life everlasting.

My cancer diagnosis certainly made me more aware of my own beliefs and faith. I found myself praying more often and asking for people's prayers. I'm not that unusual. A study of 200 elderly people in Kansas City showed that 91 percent said their initial response to a new medical problem is prayer. Prayer is frequently used as coping mechanism for dealing with serious disease.

Spirituality and healing has become more accepted in the medical community, which has traditionally not embraced the idea that faith plays a role in healing. Today more than a third of America's 125 medical schools offer "faith in healing" curricula. Despite Hawking's conclusions, we should thank God science is delving into the interplay between faith and medicine.

When it Rains, It Pours

Morton Salt's label displays a little girl holding an umbrella. The tag line on the label reads "when it rains, it pours" which was adapted from the old proverb, "it never rains, but it pours." The clever ad campaign and branding came about as a result of Morton's innovation of adding magnesium carbonate (anti-caking agent) to salt, creating a table salt that flowed freely. (That is, even when it rains, it (the salt) pours!)

The real meaning of the proverb is that something doesn't happen for a long time, and then it seems to happen all at once. Swarms and clusters happen in life. Life events are rarely evenly spaced.

Remember the year Hurricane Charley hit? Storms were coming at us one after the other that year. I was in Japan attending Yoko's mother's funeral when Charley hit. Our home was destroyed by the storm. We had to gut the house and rebuild. Since then we've been pretty lucky. Let's hope our luck continues.

It's been six years since Charley and five years since we moved back into our house. We haven't had to do much around the house for the last few years, but suddenly we've had a rash of things that need to be repaired or replaced. It's as though things know that, after five years, it's time to break.

Our household repairs this summer included the air conditioner in my daughter's car, a replacement set of tires for Yoko's car, a repair job on the freezer and ice machine, a new sewer line from the house to the street, repairs to the pool pump, the cruise control on my car, and replacing our home entertainment system. Oh well, the good news is it's nothing that can't be fixed and we are fortunate enough to be able to afford to fix the things that break!

When it comes to the human body, repairs are not so easy and the cost is not so cheap. As we age, physical problems also seem to swarm. Have you ever noticed that when you are not well, it's not just one thing?

Many people I know have had a hip or knee replacement, surgery for a bad rotator cuff, surgery to correct a bad back or other ailing parts. Many of these people are back to living an active life, without the previous pain and discomfort. Many say that, in retrospect, they wonder why they waited so long to take corrective measures. Unquestionably, medicine has made fantastic progress in my lifetime when it comes to replacing failing body parts.

A friend of mine has a 20-something year old son who developed ameloblastoma, which is a rare benign tumor that appears in the mandible. The symptoms were a "toothache" which his son ignored for some time. The tumor in his jaw was discovered after he finally visited a dentist. His son was treated last month by excising the tumor with surgery (removing all of the affected bone) and replacing a large piece of his jaw with a graft from his leg. The procedure took a team of surgeons 14 hours to complete. His son was in post-surgical intensive care for several days and is now, thankfully, on the mend. Rehabilitation will take months but he has a good prognosis for leading a completely normal life. Praise God!

In January of this year the Virginia B Andes Volunteer Community Clinic arranged for a bilateral hip replacement for a disabled patient who was wheelchair bound by bone on bone hip pain in both joints. The hospital operating room, surgeon, anesthetist, nurses, hip prosthetics, transportation, and rehabilitation services were all donated by our caring medical community. This patient is not only walking again, but he's going back to work! All things break in time, but what can be better than fixing an injured body and repairing a broken life.

Lung Cancer — The Number One Killer of Women

Three years ago my daughter Jessie was just starting her college career and Yoko and I were beginning a new life as "empty nesters." We made plans to travel. Labor Day weekend 2007 we went to visit friends in New Mexico. I remember having had a cough that would not go away, but I was convinced it was allergies. Little did I know that less than a month later I would be diagnosed with lung cancer.

Next week will mark the third anniversary of my Stage IIIA lung cancer diagnosis. My cancer was discovered in an x-ray by my primary care physician. I remember my wife asking me what the doctor had to say about my cough after coming home from my annual physical. Not yet having the test results, I jokingly told her I had lung cancer; the very next day I learned the joke was on me.

Like anyone diagnosed with cancer, my life changed that day and it will never be the same. But I did not want the remainder of my life to now be about cancer treatments and declining health. I determined to accommodate the necessary treatments, whatever came, but not be ruled by them.

For example, I did not want to make changes to our "empty nester" travel plans. Yoko and I went to visit my sister in Houston the weekend following my first round of chemo. A few weeks later, I went to radiation in the morning followed by chemo until mid-afternoon. That same day we drove to Tallahassee to see Jessie and attend a Saturday afternoon FSU football game. I wore one of those crazy garnet wigs to the game and attributed my new hair color and out of control hair style to the radiation treatments.

In those early days I was hoping to be able to attend Paula's wedding, but I didn't think I would live long enough to see Jessie's college graduation. Three years later, I am enjoying good health and looking forward to the future. Oldest daughter Paula, who is now married, is having a baby boy in February. My baby girl, Jessie, will graduate college in May.

Cancer never leaves you. Not a day goes by that I don't think about having this disease. It's incorporated into my life. It's part of who I am and what I do. I have added surviving inoperable lung cancer to my greatest accomplishments, which include mastering the Japanese language, getting Yoko to marry me, and raising and educating my three beautiful girls. These past three years of living with cancer have been some of the most fulfilling years of my life. There is still more I want to do.

October is breast cancer awareness month. The entire country will, once again, be plastered with pink thanks to the efforts of breast cancer advocates. Mark my words: women, not men, will find the cure for cancer.

I've been jealous of the attention paid to breast cancer while lung cancer — the No. 1 cancer killer of women — is practically ignored. Lung cancer remains in the shadows and on the back burner when it comes to research. No one knows why a young woman, like my friend and fellow advocate, Melissa Petersen, is suddenly cut down by lung cancer. Melissa was in the prime of her life with two small children and no history of smoking. She, like many others, believed that hormonal changes during pregnancy may have had something to do with her developing the disease.

The National Lung Cancer Partnership suggested I attend the National Breast Cancer Coalition's LEADS workshop in Minneapolis this weekend. The three-day conference will bring breast cancer advocates together to learn about the latest developments in cancer research. There's a lot I can learn from breast cancer advocates. I hope to teach them to "look deeper" too.

The Deadline to End Breast Cancer

On Thursday afternoon I flew to Minneapolis to take part in the National Breast Cancer Coalition's LEAD Project, an intensive three-day workshop designed to train breast cancer advocates. LEAD stands for leadership, education, advocacy and development. The seminar is well named. It is designed to educate and develop advocate leaders in the breast cancer movement. I attended the conference at the recommendation of The National Lung Cancer Partnership and I am glad I did.

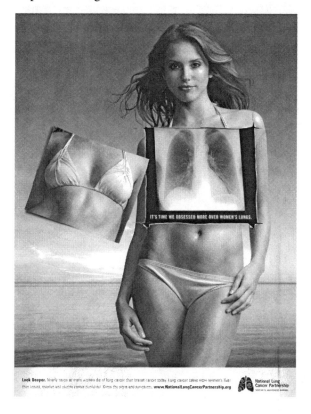

National Lung Cancer Partnership's "Look Deeper" lung cancer awareness campaign.

This time last year I was writing about "Octoberbreast," when every town in America is painted pink. As a lung cancer advocate I have been jealous of the support and funding for breast cancer as compared to lung cancer. So I was a little apprehensive about attending this conference and then saying something inappropriate. In the end, I decided that the best policy was to say as little as possible and just listen.

First, I have to say that the group assembled — both teaching staff and students — was impressive. The lecturers included cancer researchers from the National Cancer Institute and various teaching staff and physicians from such educational institutions as Virginia Tech, Harvard, Amherst College, and The University of Minnesota. The "students" included breast cancer researchers as well as advocates and organizers from the mid-West, many of whom are nurses, physicians and epidemiologists. The group was reflective of the entire country including blacks, whites, Asians and Hispanics. However, I was the only male in the class, which was really no surprise. (Every cancer conference I have been to in the last two years has been dominated by women.)

This particular group was knowledgeable, well educated, thoughtful and fun. Many were breast cancer survivors. Over the three days I learned the basics of cellular biology as it relates to cancer, some of the basics of epidemiology, and how to read and interpret medical research reports with a critical eye. I also learned about the cellular biology of the latest targeted drug therapies and how they work. The LEAD Project is renowned for training knowledgeable breast cancer advocates and I can see why.

During conference breaks and at mealtime I was able to speak with many of these women who have been through treatments very similar to mine. I was surprised to learn that we could speak the same language and that our experiences as cancer patients were not all that different. Many of the participants were not aware of lung cancer mortality rates and funding statistics. Most were surprised and open to the idea that lung cancer is as much a women's issue as breast cancer.

Many of the questions they are asking in the breast cancer movement and at this conference are the same as the questions I have: for example, why are so many young women developing breast cancer (and lung cancer)?

I was surprised to learn about the shortcomings of mammography as a screening technology and that some women have a "predisposition" to breast cancer, if they have certain gene mutations. It made me think that there may be similar gene mutations for lung cancer that have not been discovered.

It would be hard to summarize all that I learned in three days. What I can say is that I now have a better understanding of the overlapping interests of breast and lung cancer. The National Breast Cancer Coalition announced at the conference that they are setting a date for the end of breast cancer — January 1 2020. They believe setting a deadline for results will be the first step in replacing "hope" and "pink" with a plan of action. That is an idea I certainly endorse. Why not make it ALL cancers?

Somehow we have to learn what genetic predisposition results in men not becoming involved in cancer advocacy. If we can unlock that mysterious genetic code, we could redouble our efforts to end cancer.

Supporting Cancer Charities and Research Funding

I was recently nominated by the National Lung Cancer Partnership to become a grant reviewer for the Cancer Prevention and Research Institute of Texas (CPRIT). Texas is devoting $3 billion over 10 years to fund cancer research under the Texas Cancer Plan. I will learn in the next few weeks if I am selected to serve on a grant review board. I hope I am chosen as I would love to see the process by which cancer research proposals are funded.

One in four Americans will develop some form of cancer during their lifetime. We all have an interest in finding methods for cancer screening and prevention. Hopefully, by funding the right research we will one day find a cure.

According to the American Cancer Society there were 11.4 million Americans living with cancer in January, 2006, the latest year for which statistics are available. (Sadly, only 400,000 were lung cancer survivors.) More than 1.5 million Americans will be newly diagnosed with cancer in 2010. That figure does not include nearly 2 million people who will be diagnosed with basal and squamous cell skin cancers.

All of us should feel some obligation to support a cancer charity, if not for ourselves, than for someone we love. There are many charities to choose from.

By far the largest and wealthiest cancer charity in the US is the American Cancer Society (ACS). In 2009 the ACS received more than $756 million in revenues from all sources. "Relay for Life" and other special events accounted for more than half the ACS's annual funding, raising over $455 million nationwide. At the end of 2009, the charity's balance sheet had $984 million in cash assets and more than $2 billion in net assets.

According to its latest annual report ACS spent about $732 million in program services in 2009, including $150 million for cancer research, $177 million for prevention and education, $129 million for detection and treatment, and $275 million for patient support. Roughly $62 million was spent on executive and administrative overhead and $222 million was used for fundraising to "secure charitable financial support." Of the $150 million ACS spent on research only $14 million was directly related to lung cancer.

The second largest cancer charity in the US is Susan G. Komen for the Cure. Over the last 30 years it has had remarkable success in marketing the breast cancer cause and attracting corporate sponsorships and donations. The large number of breast cancer survivors and advocates, most of whom are older women, makes this an attractive market for companies to support.

Komen's 2009 annual report boasts of more than 240 corporate partners, including Conde Nast publications, which last year sponsored 3,500 golf, tennis and dining events, American Airlines "Miles for the Cure" program, Bank of America's "Pink Ribbon Banking" program, Ford's "Race for the Cure", General Mills' "Pink Together" program, and so on.

In 2009 Komen raised a total of $346 million and spent $276 million on program services. About $60 million was used for breast cancer research, according to its annual report. Komen's administrative overhead amounted to $66 million, including $39 million for general administration and $29 million for fundraising.

Another charity fighting for cancer dollars, and the one that I naturally favor, is the National Lung Cancer Partnership, which is specifically devoted to raising money for lung cancer research. This year the Partnership's "Free to Breathe" branded events organized nationwide by a small cadre of survivor volunteers are expected to raise a meager $2.5 million.

State of Emotions: What's next?

Tonight I came home from another busy day, turned on the TV and started watching "The Biggest Looser." It is not something I normally watch, but I am fascinated by how the show creates drama and emotion. If you think about it, a bunch of overweight people trying to lose weight should not be the stuff of high drama. Yet somehow the show titillates and keeps you engaged by implicitly asking "what happens next?" That question is what keeps life interesting in general.

Last week at this time Yoko and I were watching the election returns. We were not surprised at the outcome. The people were speaking and you would have to be hard of hearing not to understand what they were saying. Still, we're looking forward to seeing what happens next. Every day a little bit more of the unfolding political drama is revealed. I love it!

I think a lot about how lucky I am to be alive to enjoy life's happenings. I appreciate mundane everyday things more than I ever did. On my daily morning walks with the dog I think about the wonder of nature and how incredibly improbable life is. Life will come to an end for us all — one way or another. But what a gift we have to be alive and conscious and wondering every day, what happens next!

Yoko and I went north over the weekend to participate in the Free to Breathe 5K Run/Walk in Ponte Vedra Beach organized by my friend and fellow survivor, Julia Stroud. They had over 800 participants and raised more than $130,000 for lung cancer research. Julia was overcome with emotion as she addressed the crowd, including our friend Mary, a Stage IV survivor now battling multiple metastases to the brain. Mary's having a hard time as do many lung cancer patients as they near the end stages of the disease. I share Julia's emotion.

After we returned from Jacksonville I received a moving letter from a woman who's been reading my newspaper column each week. Her father, a WWII veteran, fought a three-year battle with lung cancer and lost six years ago. She's not gotten over her loss. Her description of the pain and suffering he endured brought tears to my eyes. No one should have to endure such indignities.

I've been collecting the names of people who have died of lung cancer — residents, friends or relatives of people who live in Charlotte County. Sadly I have over 70 signs to be displayed at this year's "Mile of Memories" walk. I attended the Board of County Commissioner's meeting to receive a proclamation declaring November 13 Lung Cancer Awareness Day. As the proclamation was read, I thought of all the people I know personally who are fighting this disease and became unexpectedly emotional.

Advocating for lung cancer lead me to writing to NBC Nightly News at the end of October when on a single news broadcast it had two lengthy stories about the fight against breast cancer. I wrote to complain bitterly that in 10 years I had not seen a single story on lung cancer, the No. 1 cancer killer. To my surprise, Robert Bazell, the Chief Health and Science Correspondent for NBC News, replied immediately. My complaint apparently got his attention. He said that he alone had done 24 stories in the past five years. He acknowledged that "one could argue that 24 stories in five year are not enough for the number one cancer killer." I agree.

Call it coincidence, but two days later NBC Nightly News' top story was about the results of a clinical trial showing that low-dose CT scan may offer a clinically acceptable way to screen for lung cancer. That's a real breakthrough — both the trial results and the news story. I'll be curious to see what happens next.

Delving Deeper into Cancer Research

In 2007 voters in the State of Texas overwhelmingly approved a resolution to issue $3 billion in bonds to fund groundbreaking cancer research and prevention programs and services in Texas over a 10-year period. The voter's approval resulted in the birth of the Cancer Prevention and Research Institute of Texas, better known as CPRIT, whose mission is to expedite innovation and commercialization in the area of cancer research and enhance access to evidence-based prevention programs and services throughout the state. Texas voters are pretty smart and we here in Florida could take a page or two from the lessons they are teaching.

The first goal of CPRIT is to create and expedite innovative research and make Texas a kind of Mecca for cancer research. This is going to attract and expand research capabilities of both public and private institutions and create a significant number of high quality new jobs in the state.

Well, yahoo! What a great idea! Invest in cancer research, create high quality jobs, and couple that with promoting prevention and healthy lifestyles. The Texas Cancer Plan will ultimately return dividends in the form of lowered healthcare costs. That all seems like it makes good sense. Why couldn't we do the same thing here in Florida?

Not too long ago I was contacted by the National Lung Cancer Partnership to see if I would be interested in representing the Partnership as a patient advocate for CPRIT. Texas law requires that committees judging grant applications must be composed of people from outside the state. Furthermore, the panels must include not only scientists, but also advocates to give voice to cancer patients. Of course, I was glad to have the opportunity and accepted the nomination — like I don't have enough to do already!

Last week I attended the first CPRIT conference in Austin. This was a gathering of researchers and grant applicants from across the state. There was an exhibit hall at the Austin Conference Center, where the event was held, filled with poster abstracts depicting research projects both proposed and funded with CPRIT grant money. The display was not unlike a high school science fair, but the science being displayed was so high level and so far beyond my meager understanding it might as well have been written in Chinese.

At the plenary sessions they had world renowned scientists and researchers discussing such topics as "Gene and Pathways that Prevent Genome Instability — from Model Organisms to Cancer Genetics." Nobel Laureate Dr. Phil Sharp was a keynote speaker at lunch discussing the topic of "Investing and Treating Cancer with RNA." It was all Greek to me!

One of the best presentations of the conference (that I could actually understand) was by Don Listwin, a former Cisco Systems top executive and founder of the Canary Foundation, named after the idea of a canary in a coal mine. His topic was "A Comprehensive Research Model for the Early Detection of Cancer."

Don lost his mother to misdiagnosed ovarian cancer. He discovered that although almost $10 billion is spent annually on cancer research in the United States, the vast majority is allocated to developing new cancer treatments and caring for patients. Surprisingly, little funding is available to investigate new ways to detect cancer at its earliest, curable stages.

Don's idea is to create simple, low cost blood tests or use molecular imaging diagnostics to detect trace amounts of proteins called biomarkers, produced by cancer. The scientific team lead by Nobel Laureate Dr. Lee Hartwell initially focused on ovarian cancer, which, like lung cancer, is asymptomatic until it is late stage. It was encouraging to learn that the scientific team has made good progress and is now moving to clinical trials for ovarian, prostate and lung cancer. That's really good news for all of us.

Making the Hard Choices

It seems like when I am not working I am doing something related to cancer. A couple of weeks ago it was the Free to Breathe 5K Run/Walk to raise money for lung cancer research. My ongoing work for the National Lung Cancer Partnership occupies a lot of my spare time. The week before Thanksgiving I was in Texas for the CPRIT (Cancer Prevention Research Institute of Texas) conference, where I learned about new technology being developed to treat various forms of cancer.

This week I have been reviewing grant proposals for CPRIT. The applications I was assigned to critique all have to do with measures to reduce the mortality of cancer by improving detection among poor, medically underserved populations. Our job on the review panel is to decide what proposals we recommend be funded. It's not going to be easy to choose between many worthwhile projects.

Each grant application is 40 to 60 pages in length describing the project to be funded, the timeline for implementation, the expected outcome and benefits and the requested dollars and justification. As Board Chair of the Virginia B Andes Volunteer Community Clinic, I know how much time and effort is required to put a grant proposal together and how important grant funding is to sustaining non-profit organizations. That makes choosing among the many applicants all the more difficult.

I was assigned ten grant proposals to review and critique. I finally completed my assignments over the holiday weekend but I have to say I struggled to rate the applications and rank them. They were all good.

Most of the grant requests I reviewed seek to fund outreach programs aimed at increasing screening for cervical, colorectal or breast cancer. The target populations were for the most part the uninsured rural poor, who have little or no access to healthcare services. These populations have relatively high cancer incidence and mortality rates compared to the general population. A common thread in nearly all the proposals was the need to educate the target population about healthy lifestyles — diet and exercise — as well as about screening.

Reading these proposals it occurred to me that health education that brings about behavioral change is probably the single most important thing we can do to fight cancer and improve the health of our nation and our economic future. Unhealthy lifestyle choices translate into higher incidence of disease and skyrocketing healthcare costs, sapping our economic strength. That is not exactly news. But if we want to make the world a better place, we need to start with ourselves by making healthy choices and investing in wellness.

Knowing what we should do is not the same as DOING what we should do. What we need as a nation is behavioral change. I'm talking about working on losing weight and keeping our body mass index to less than 25. It means giving up cigarettes, reducing our alcohol intake and foregoing super-sized meals. It means getting outside to exercise and using sunscreen religiously when we do. It means, in short, changing our behavior and making the right choices in our daily lives. It's easier said than done. What we all need is some motivation.

I was in my convertible driving around town the other day when I smelled cigarette smoke spewing from a vehicle next to me. It's bad enough to see cigarette addicted young people risking their own health; what was worse was seeing these parents risk the health of their children in the back. I resisted saying anything to these young parents, but it occurred to me that there should be a law or ordinance on the books that would allow the police to fine this kind of reckless child endangerment.

Maybe public policy needs to motivate people to make healthy choices with fines, surcharges and tax incentives. Hitting people in the wallet will usually get their attention.

A Joyous Season Begins

I had a PET and CT scan today at Advanced Imaging to see if I am still in remission. Six months is the longest I have gone, so far, without a scan since my diagnosis in October of 2007.

Today's test was much less intimidating than when I first had to go. Of course, I now know what to expect and the folks at Advanced Imaging have gotten to know me as well. They are prepared for my quirky needs. I get claustrophobic in the machine, for example, so they give me a sedative when I first arrive to help take the edge off. They allow me to wear my I-pod during the test. (I programmed it with a 30 minute playlist so I could keep track of time while inside the scanner.) Between the sedative and soothing music, I didn't experience the claustrophobic fear I felt on previous exams.

After the test was over I was invited back to review the images with Dr. Fabian. (I did not want to leave the place not knowing whether I remain cancer free or not so I asked if we could review the scans together.) There was nothing new to be observed in the pictures and there was no evidence of disease. What a great way to begin the joyous season! Thank you Jesus!

I feel like a man released from prison, if only on probation. I can stay free to live my life at least until the next exam.

This is especially good news because we're getting ready for a special Christmas family reunion — a ski vacation this year in

Colorado, which has been planned for some time. It's a relief to know that cancer, at least, won't be interfering.

I'm reading a book entitled "The Emperor of All Maladies — A Biography of Cancer" written by Siddhartha Mukherjee. It is a very well written account of the history of cancer research and treatment.

The prologue describes how the author and six other oncology fellows at the National Cancer Institute felt that "cancer was an all-consuming presence in our lives. It invaded our imaginations; it occupied our memories; it infiltrated every conversation, every thought. And if we, as physicians, found ourselves immersed in cancer, then our patients found their lives virtually obliterated by the disease."

That description really struck me. Since diagnosis I feel as though cancer has consumed and redefined my life. Even though I am now in remission it has come to define who I am in the same way a veteran is defined by the war in which he or she served.

I know many cancer patients struggling with different forms of this disease. I feel the guilt of a survivor who lives to fight another day while others die. More needs to be done to save the many precious lives being lost to this disease.

In 1985 a Harvard biologist named John Cairns wrote that "the death rate from malaria, cholera, typhus, tuberculosis; scurvy, pellagra and other scourges of the past have dwindled in the US because we have learned how to prevent these diseases. To put most of the (cancer) effort into treatment (rather than prevention) is to deny all precedent." I agree. Much more research into cancer prevention is needed.

This Christmas season I give God special thanks for allowing me to live.

Marking the Passage of Time

Every Christmas for the past 23 years I have written a Christmas letter documenting the progress our family has made from year to year. I put a lot of effort into writing these annual Christmas missives, which I have tried to make both informative and entertaining. Yoko and I have saved most of the letters going back to 1987 and they are fun to re-read every year. We sure have come a long way since those days!

I remember the first major purchase I made after graduating from college in 1978. I was working for a major Japanese trading company in Tokyo living in a company dorm at no cost and earning a salary of $12,000 a year. With virtually no living expenses, I saved enough to buy a high-end stereo system — a Sony solid-state tuner and amplifier, cassette tape player and turntable, wood cabinet and large floor speakers. I don't remember what I spent, but it wasn't cheap.

Four years later, after I was married and Paula was born, we moved back to the States. The Sony system didn't work in the US without a transformer and the tuner bandwidth was different in the US. By that time the world was starting to move to CDs and my "high end" stereo was fast becoming obsolete. As we prepared to move back to Japan in 1986 I sold the whole kit and caboodle for a few hundred bucks.

I bought my first car in 1982. It was a used 1973 Ford Maverick stick-shift with manual steering and about 100,000 miles on it. I remember the car cost about $1,200, which was 20% of my savings at the time. I was 28 with a wife and baby and $5,000 to my name and no income. We owned that car for two years while I was in grad school living on borrowed money. I never had to repair it or put money into it, so I guess it was a pretty good deal. I think we sold it for 600 bucks when we moved to California two years later.

The first time I wrote a computer generated Christmas letter was in 1987 after purchasing a state of the art IBM PS2 and a Hewlett Packard laser printer, together with a VGA monitor and graphic card. I was living in Japan again and ordered the system from Chicago. I had it shipped to our home in Tokyo and I distinctly remember the total cost, door to door, being a heart-stopping sum of $13,000, more than my annual salary five years earlier. It also required a bulky transformer to work in Japan and came with no warranty outside the US.

The PS2 ran on a 286 Intel chip and had a 40mb hard disk drive. It used a 3.5 inch floppy disk drive for external storage and initially ran on the DOS 3.0 operating system. The PS2 was state of the art at the time I bought it. I could not imagine how I would ever use the massive 40 megabyte hard drive until Windows came along. Back then I was definitely considered a "power user" and early adopter.

I remember my parents visiting us in Tokyo that Christmas. My father, who was quite frugal and technology illiterate, questioned my need for a personal computer. Who would spend that kind of money just to balance a checkbook or write a letter?

Since that first Christmas letter we have chronicled my girls growing up. Our world has changed.

I am now an expectant grandfather, close to the same age my father was when he visited us in Japan more than two decades ago. I'm beginning to understand "the circle of life" as I struggle not to become obsolete myself.

Still, I have to wonder …who could possibly need the 64 gigs of storage in an iPad?

Part V — 2011

Don't Tread on Me

In the movie *Network* there was a scene where a frustrated New York tenant angrily yells out from his apartment window, "I'm mad as hell and I'm not going to take it anymore!" We all know the feeling. Modern life can be infuriating and sometimes it makes you want to strike back.

Our forefathers felt a similar frustration with British rule. In return for Britain's exporting convicts to America, Ben Franklin, famed for his satirical humor, suggested we return the favor by sending rattlesnakes to England. The rattlesnake evolved into a symbol of unity and freedom and was famously incorporated into the Gadsden flag, with the words, "Don't Tread on Me". The unstated threat is "Or Else."

So, what's gotten me so hot under the collar? I've been bitten by snakes and it makes me want to strike back. Here's what happened:

I learned that the traveling Broadway production of "South Pacific" was being performed at the Barbara B. Mann Center for Performing Arts Hall in Fort Myers. It's one of my favorite musicals and I have not seen a Broadway production in many years, so we decided to go.

I googled the term "Barbara B. Mann," found the theater website at the top of the list (or so I thought), clicked on the "buy tickets" link, and purchased two tickets on the "Tickets Now" website. I promptly received the tickets by Federal Express and put them aside for the night of the event.

I naturally thought I had made the purchase from a legitimate ticket vendor affiliated with Barbara B. Mann. The tickets were $88 each, which was expensive, but it appeared that the show was nearly sold out and I assumed that the price I paid was the going price for more expensive premium seating. That was my mistake. I should have taken more time and looked more closely.

Including service charges, the tickets I received in the mail cost a total of $236 — the most I have ever paid for theater tickets in Florida — but I was willing to pay for what I thought were good seats.

When we got to the theater on Saturday, I finally opened the envelope and looked at the tickets. To my surprise the tickets had a $43 face value. Worse, after we entered the hall, we found our seats in the nose bleed section, where you need oxygen to breathe and opera glasses to see. That's when I realized I had been electronically mugged.

I called the vendor, Tickets Now, to complain and learned for the first time that I had made the purchase from a ticket reseller who is not affiliated with Barbara B. Mann. Their basic stance is "buyers beware." They claim the nature of their service is disclosed on their website. If there was any disclosure, I never saw it. Naturally, they don't disclose the face value of what you are buying!

The next call I made was to Barbara B Mann's box office manager. They know about scam websites reselling tickets, but the manager claims that there is nothing they can do about unsavory resellers, who, in Florida, freely function as electronic scalpers. The theater has tried to deal with this problem without success. The business is not regulated in Florida.

I asked the box office manager if they sell blocks of tickets to resellers and he said they don't. Their policy is to sell no more than eight tickets to any one party. Nevertheless, somehow, Tickets Now gets product for resale.

It's my understanding that resellers are able to purchase from Google the top spots for certain search term results. They stay at the top of the list until they get a predetermined number of clicks. If that's true, Google, in effect, facilitates the scam by presenting misleading search results. Isn't that fraud?

Making Cancer a Rare Disease Again

Since my diagnosis of lung cancer in 2007, I have read everything I can about the disease. I've tried to become educated and knowledgeable about cancer in general and lung cancer in particular. What I have learned is that the disease called "cancer" is so broad and encompassing that the term is rendered nearly meaningless. I have also learned that the variety of cancers –particularly the anomalies of rare cancers — is what has given scientists the greatest insights to the workings of the disease.

Cancer has a long history. The word first appeared in 400 BC, around the time of Hippocrates. It comes from the Greek word "Karkinos" meaning crab. But cancer was described in detail as far back as 2665 BC by an Egyptian physician named Imhotep. While cancer was known by the ancients it was not a leading cause of death. Cancer has only come to the fore in the 20th century.

I always thought the proliferation of carcinogens in our environment was the root cause of the modern cancer epidemic. In fact, the reason that cancer today is no longer the rare disease that it once was is because of the fantastic progress we have made in treating other diseases.

In the past people died relatively young from diseases such as smallpox, tuberculosis, polio, malaria, typhoid fever, and a host of other maladies. Today these once common ailments are rare diseases in the United States. The advent of vaccines and antibiotics in the last century reduced deaths from these causes.

Cancer typically develops over time as people age. Thanks to the progress of modern science, longer life expectancy in the developed world makes cancer more prominent as a disease and leading cause of death.

Cancer is a disease that can be triggered by carcinogens, but what we now know is that cancer is essentially genetic in nature. That discovery was made by studying the rarer forms of cancer.

The story of a 19th century Brazilian ophthalmologist, who documented treating a patient with a rare eye cancer called a retinoblastoma, is a case in point. The patient was treated by removing the eye. The young boy survived his cancer. He eventually married a woman with no history of cancer. The couple had several children and two of the daughters developed retinoblastoma in both eyes and died of the disease. The case strongly suggested to scientists in the 20th century that an inherited factor lived in genes that caused cancer.

We now know that cancer is a disease of uncontrolled growth of a single cell related to malignant genes. The best description or explanation I have heard is that cancer is like a speeding car with a stuck accelerator (resulting in quickly multiplying cells) and no brakes (no cell death or "apoptosis"). Finding the genetic cause of a rare childhood disease — retinoblastoma — became the focus of MD Andersen researcher Alfred Kundson, who, in 1969, postulated the existence of oncogenes and anti-oncogenes — the genetic gas pedals and breaks of cancer cells.

Genetic malignancies either inherited or triggered by carcinogens, give rise to cancer. The key to curing the disease, therefore, is to find ways to stop malignant cells from forming in the first place, inhibiting their multiplication or causing them to die.

Leukemia, which is a cancer of the blood or bone marrow, is characterized by an overabundance of malignant white blood cells. It was a cancer that was at one time untreatable. Sidney Farber, known as the father of chemotherapy, learned how long-term survivors of the mustard gas attack at Ypres during World War I were observed to have become anemic, requiring blood transfusions. Farber put two and two together and discovered that chemicals could be used to target leukemia.

Thanks to research, progress is being made to make cancer a rare disease once again

"God Winks" Galore

I belong to a small prayer group that meets once a month to talk about matters of faith and religion. The group, which is non-sectarian, was organized by my friend Janet and her husband Bill.

Janet named the group "God Winks" as a reference to the idea that God shows Himself every day in our daily life, but we don't always recognize His hand in things. From time to time a light goes off and we can see divine intervention.

At each meeting of God Winks we start with a prayer and reading from the writings of Joel Osteen, a prominent Christian minister. The reading usually leads to some discussion of what has happened in the last month and the "God Winks" we have experienced.

At last week's meeting I related how I had run into a member of our prayer group at the Atlanta airport just as we were about to board the plane to Fort Myers. The flight had been delayed three hours and was going to be arriving very late. It turned out this person needed a ride home and was thinking about how she was going to get home from her late-night arrival when I miraculously appeared and plopped myself directly in front of her. I was literally the answer to her prayers that evening! You might call this a happy coincidence, but in our group we call it a God Wink.

I am writing about "God Winks" this week because there has been a cornucopia of coincidences in my life in recent days.

The latest wink involves a fellow named Pete, who was diagnosed with cancer. I learned about Pete's story from a client of mine who thought I would be interested in writing about his story for the newspaper.

Pete is a sixty-something year-old man who was diagnosed with pancreatic cancer earlier this year. He was showing severe symptoms, including urine that was black and signs of jaundice. He was passed from one doctor to another, at first here locally and eventually at Tampa General. It wasn't too long before Pete and his wife got the bad news. He had inoperable pancreatic cancer and there was nothing really they could do because the tumor's proximity to the portal artery made surgery impossible.

The doctor who delivered the bad news decided to do one more scan. In the meantime, Pete and his wife researched surgeons and found a doctor, who happened to be at Tampa General. This doctor specializes in surgical treatment of pancreatic cancer, performing about 150 pancreatic cancer surgeries a year.

Pete consulted with the specialist who decided that he could do the surgery after all, with the proviso that there was no guarantee that Pete would even survive the operation.

With no other alternative, Pete went ahead and underwent an extensive surgery on April 5, which removed his gall bladder, part of his intestine and a portion of his pancreas. When the pathology came back, post surgery, Pete learned that the tumor was benign, which occurs only in about 4 percent of pancreatic cancer cases.

Pete says he learned three things from this experience: the power of prayer; that miracles do happen, and the value of getting a second opinion. He is on the mend and can look forward to a full recovery.

Now here is the God Wink; Pete is friends with a woman I helped through the Virginia B Andes clinic obtain surgical treatment for lung cancer.

A Recipe for Handling Adversity

A friend of mine sent me this little story of inspiration. It is something to be taken to heart by anyone facing adversity!

Carrot, Egg and Coffee...

Author Unknown

A young woman went to her mother and complained about life and how things were so hard for her. She did not know how she was going to make it and wanted to give up. She was tired of the everyday fighting and struggling. It seemed that when one problem was solved, a new one arose.

Her mother beckoned her into the kitchen and boiled three pots of water. In the first she placed carrots, in the second she placed eggs, and in the last she placed ground coffee beans.

She let them all boil for a while without saying a word. In time she turned off the burners and fished out the carrots, eggs and coffee, placing each in a separate bowl. Turning to her daughter, she asked, "Tell me what you see." "Carrots, eggs, and coffee," the daughter replied.

Her mother brought her closer and asked her to feel the carrots. She did and noted that they were soft. The mother then asked the daughter to take an egg and break it. After pulling off the shell, she observed the hard-boiled egg. Finally, the mother asked the daughter to sip the coffee. The daughter smiled as she tasted its flavor and smelled the rich aroma. The daughter then asked, "What is your point, mother?"

Her mother explained how each of these objects had faced the same adversity — boiling water. Each reacted differently. The carrot went in strong, hard, and unrelenting. However, after being subjected to the boiling water, it softened and became weak. The egg had been fragile. Its thin outer shell had protected its liquid interior, but after sitting through the boiling water, its inside became hardened. But the ground coffee beans subjected to boiling water had changed the water itself. "Which are you?" she asked her daughter. "When adversity knocks on your door, how do you respond? Are you a carrot, an egg or a coffee bean?"

Am I the carrot that seems strong, but with pain and adversity do I wilt and become soft and lose my strength?

Am I the egg that starts with a malleable heart, but changes with the heat? Did I have a fluid spirit, but after a death, a breakup, a financial hardship or some other trial, have I become hardened and stiff? Does my shell look the same, but on the inside am I bitter and tough with a stiff spirit and hardened heart?

Or am I like the coffee bean that changes the hot water, the very circumstance that brings the pain? When the water gets hot, it releases its fragrance and flavor.

If you are like the bean, when things are at their worst, you get better and change the situation around you. When the hour is the darkest and trials are their greatest, do you elevate yourself to another level? How do you handle adversity? Are you a carrot, an egg or a coffee bean?

May you have enough happiness to make you sweet, enough trials to make you strong, enough sorrow to keep you human and enough hope to make you happy. The happiest people don't necessarily have the best of everything; they just make the most of everything that comes their way.

The brightest future will always be based on a forgotten past; you can't go forward in life until you let go of your past failures and heart aches. When you were born, you were crying and everyone around you was smiling. Live your life so at the end, you're the one who is smiling and everyone around you is crying.

Civility, Decency, Dignity and Decorum

Anyone who knows me knows that I am not confrontational or combative. I've never struck anyone in anger. I don't call people derogatory names. I don't provoke arguments. I've never owned a gun and I wouldn't want to have one. When I disagree with someone, I try to persuade them to my way of thinking, but I don't berate them if they don't happen to see things my way.

I am very much for freedom, particularly freedom of speech. Toleration of extreme views (on either the left or the right) is a small price to pay for that freedom. My attitude is "to each his own" provided it does not intrude on my freedom. I believe citizens have responsibilities (to society) as well as rights (as individuals). However I think it is a mistake to talk about rights without also referencing responsibility. It should be a matched pair. For example, all citizens should have an absolute right to vote, but they should also be responsible for being educated about the issues! That's not something we can legislate but it is something that would make our democracy work a lot better.

I believe in social justice and fairness, but I don't believe in a welfare state that creates dependents. Government cannot be the only solution to our problems. At the end of the day, we have to look to ourselves and the individual roles we play. We all need to be part of the solution and avoid becoming part of the problem. In a nutshell, democracy starts with me. I am responsible for my own actions or inaction. It's why I am fighting for the tens of thousands of lung cancer victims who are anonymously dying every day.

The assassination attempt on Representative Gabriel Gifford in Tucson last week has been on the news 24/7 for more than a week now. The shooting massacre by a clearly deranged killer has somehow morphed into a national debate about our society and civility. The debate, in part, is over whether political rhetoric and partisan bickering influenced the thinking of an insane killer in Arizona. As a nation we seemed to have latched onto this event as somehow reflecting our collective national character. It has sparked a debate about being a civil society. I agree with President Obama that it is time to change the tone of our political rhetoric. If the tragedy in Arizona helps to accomplish that, then something good will have come from this awful event.

Whether or not the political environment gave rise to the rampage in Arizona, there is nothing wrong with the idea that we need to be more civil and respectful in our interaction with each other. At some point we have to get past name calling and bickering and start to debate issues on the merit without trying to spin the facts one way or the other or characterize people, who happen to disagree, as the incarnation of evil.

Diversity means that we all see the world through a different prism of experience and knowledge. We have to end divisiveness and start to sincerely listen to one another rather than talking over one another. Debate is not a contest of who can shout the loudest. Civility and decency has to start with our political leaders. I think the president was right to highlight this idea in his remarks at a memorial service for the victims last week.

I only wish he had expanded the theme to include dignity and decorum. To be honest, I thought the hooting and hollering at the Tucson memorial service was beyond the pale of being disrespectful. We can hoot and holler at a football game or rodeo, but should there be shouting and raucous whistling on a somber occasion marking the death of six people? I don't think so.

Relationships That Matter

Over the weekend I watched the movie *The Social Network*, which is about how young computer-nerd Mark Zuckerberg came to create Facebook. I found it ironic that "the social network" was created by someone portrayed in the movie as a condescending snob, who is both deceitful and socially inept. The irony is that "social networks" have somehow succeeded as a substitute for face to face social interaction, in the same way that video games have undermined physical exercise.

What are called "relationships" these days are more like cold connections. Just because I knew you 40 years ago in junior high school doesn't mean we are "friends" as a result of reconnecting through the Internet. For me, healthy relationships are in the flesh, person to person connections with people you really care about. Relationships are fragile and work only if you work on them. They have to be nurtured and maintained. Quality relationships are about the people who are the constants in your life, in good times and in bad. Your family plays the lead role; friends are the supporting actors.

I'm lucky enough to have some great relationships in my life, starting with a deep and abiding love for my wife and family and a few life-long friends. These are the people for whom I would gladly sacrifice my own life. They are the people who love me as much as I love them. The people with whom I have a real relationship know me well. They know my many faults and still see past them. The relationships that have lasted in my life are based on trust, respect and, most important, forgiveness. None of us are perfect so we have to be able to forgive.

Yoko and I will soon celebrate 30 years of marriage. I would not be honest if I didn't confess that we have had, at times, our share of difficulties. All marriages do. You don't really know someone until you've lived with them. And if you live with someone long enough, they eventually say or do something to undermine the relationship.

That is why, before entering into a committed relationship with another person, you make a vow — a solemn promise before God — to stay together for better or for worse, for richer or for poorer, in sickness and in health. Vows before God help get you through the hard times, which invariably come. You keep love's promise by nurturing your relationships. Forgiveness is weeding in the garden of love.

I've had difficulties in my life, with a diagnosis of late-stage lung cancer at the top of the list. If there was a silver lining in going through hard times, it was to understand who really cares about me, the value of a strong family and the meaning of true friendship. The joy of living is the quality relationships we have with people we love.

One of my favorite television programs is "Parenthood," now in its second season on NBC. The story centers on the lives and relationships within a family. These include the grandfather who is estranged from his wife because of infidelity, a divorced daughter raising two teenaged children alone and struggling to make ends meet, an eldest son trying to balance work and a challenging family life, and a free-spirited younger son who is coming to terms with an unplanned fatherhood. The program is appealing in the way it encapsulates the stresses and strains of maintaining quality relationships. Lord knows it isn't easy.

In "Simple Love" Allison Krauss sings about a man who lives a life devoted to his wife and daughters. The refrain of the song is, "I want a simple life like that, always giving, never asking back. And when I'm in my final hour looking back, I hope I have a simple love like that." Amen!

New Milestones and No Time to Waste

October will mark four years since I was diagnosed with inoperable Stage IIIA lung cancer. I frankly never thought I would live this long. I remember visiting my daughter Jessica at FSU in the fall of 2007 thinking I might not see her graduate. I'll never forget her tears and emotion when we talked about the possibility.

Faced with what is a terminal diagnosis, I remember thinking that I had wasted a lot of time in my life. I decided not to waste any more and got busy. Now I've made a habit of cramming as much into every hour, day, and week as I possibly can. I sometimes feel like a juggler with one too many pins in the air.

These days what I've been juggling is my schedule. I've noticed that whenever I make plans to go somewhere or do something it is almost a certainty that I'm going to be stressed for time. It's not that I procrastinate. I simply have a lot of things going on at once. I have to funnel all my commitments through a finite window of time and invariably there are conflicts. I strive to always complete the things I've committed to do on time, but that does not come without some considerable stress and strain. These last few months have been particularly difficult as I have had one family thing after another occupying my weekends.

Since mid-April I've had to go to Pennsylvania to see my elderly mother, attend my daughter's graduation in Tallahassee (a big milestone for both her and me), fly to California to visit our oldest daughter and meet our new grandson, Maddox, and then go on to Las Vegas to celebrate our 30th wedding anniversary. I'm elated to be able to have lived to see three huge milestones in my life. I hope to see more.

Right now I'm in Las Vegas for the second time this month to play in a pro-am golf tournament, which I committed to back in March. When I accepted the invitation I did not realize it would conflict with my commitment as a peer reviewer for the Cancer Prevention and Research Institute of Texas. My grant critiques are due by tomorrow, midnight, and I have two left to do. Each proposal is 60 or so pages to read and each critique takes two to three hours to write. I've known about the deadline for getting this done for over a month. The problem is finding the 20 or 30 hours to do it. Thankfully the work can be done online and the iPad Yoko gave me allows me to use the crevices between blocks of time on my busy schedule to get it done.

When I'm home I've had to write my newspaper columns, carry out my responsibilities for the Andes Volunteer Clinic and Rotary, work on projects for the National Lung Cancer Partnership, as well as attend to the needs of my clients.

Thanks to mobile technology, I am never out of touch when traveling. I know what is going on at work and in the markets via the Blackberry. I can take my iPad anywhere and be able to stay in touch and get things done. Mobile technology has been a tremendous boost to helping me get the most out of the time I have. Four years ago, the iPad was a mere apple in Steven Jobs' eye. I'm sure glad he and I both lived to see it!

Now that I've witnessed my youngest daughter, Jessica, graduate from college, I'm thinking about some new milestones and the things I hope to achieve. Next on the list is shooting a par round of golf, starting tomorrow.

Tentative Summer Plans

This Friday I have scheduled my six-month check-up to see if I am still "stable" with no evidence of disease. I will undergo a CT scan and a PET scan at Advanced Imaging, as I have done so many times before. In fact, I've lost count of how many times I have undergone these tests, but I still get anxious as the date approaches. Depending on the outcome, my life could once again be turned upside down and our plans put on hold. It's no wonder cancer patients get "scanxiety!"

I am a little more anxious this time for a couple of reasons. First, the maintenance trial drug I have been on for 30 months showed that, in the Phase II trial, the drug worked for as long as 36 months before there were signs of disease progression. I am only six months away from that outside mark. If I am going to have a recurrence, it should happen soon. The longer I go without a recurrence, the better off I am.

The second reason I am more anxious this time are the recent aches and pains that have developed in my spine and shoulder blades. I've also been experiencing cramps in my back, just beneath the shoulder blades. My original lung tumor was in the upper right posterior lobe, roughly in the spot where I am now experiencing cramps. The pain or stiffness in my spine feels like it could just be a touch of arthritis. Nevertheless, it worries me because lung cancer commonly metastasizes to the bone.

The scans on Friday will determine whether I continue to live life as usual or not. I'm praying for a good outcome and still making plans for the summer and beyond.

Over Memorial Day weekend I spoke with Yoko about travel plans for the rest of the year. What touched off the conversation was my daughter June calling to say that she and eldest daughter Paula are coming to Florida for Thanksgiving. Paula and her husband Brian would come with grandson, Maddox. June would bring her boyfriend, Will. Youngest daughter Jessica may or not be living at home by Thanksgiving, depending upon how her job search goes, but she would more than likely join us with her boyfriend. I hope it happens. It would be the first time we would all be together for Thanksgiving in years.

I've been invited by my good friend and golfing buddy, Chris Maher, to play in the ATT National Pro-Am at Aronimink Golf Club in Philadelphia at the end of June. I'm really excited about this once-in-a-lifetime chance to play a practice round with PGA touring professionals. Between now and then I need to be working on my short game!

As it so happens, my 88 year old mother, who lives in Pennsylvania, not far from Aronimink, called this weekend to inform us that she has decided it's time to move into an assisted living facility.

She plans to make the move as early as July, so I hope to take the opportunity to see her and do what I can to help her and my sister.

Yoko and I were hoping to go up to Virginia in July to see my sister, Jane, at her lakeside home. We also have the wedding of my niece to attend in Pittsburgh in August. Our other travel ambitions this year include getting down to Miami for a weekend to see friends, going to New Mexico again Labor Day weekend, and heading for Key West in October.

The only thing standing in the way of all these plans is having a clean bill of health. Assuming my good fortune holds and the scans this week come back negative, we can start moving forward with our travel plans for the rest of this year.

Cancer News Offers New Hope and New Questions

In case you hadn't noticed, this entire week has been filled with news stories about cancer and research breakthroughs. The deluge of cancer news has largely to do with the clinical research being presented at the annual ASCO (The American Society of Clinical Oncology) Convention that has been taking place in Chicago June 3 thru June 7.

The American Cancer Society deemed Monday, June 5, "Cancer Survivor Day" celebrating the continuing lives of millions of cancer survivors. Given the progress being made by cancer researchers in treating the disease, the number of cancer survivors is only going to grow.

I was encouraged by the news coming out of ASCO. Among the featured developments was a new drug from Roche, Vermurafenib, and Daiichi Sankyo's Plexxikon, both designed to treat patients with melanoma who have a certain mutation in a gene known as BRAF. Studies show that these new drugs are extending time to progression of the disease for those with a specific genetic mutation.

Another drug for advanced melanoma from Bristol Myers Squibb, Yervoy, was approved by the FDA and is already on the market. The drug is said to work on the immune system. In combination with other chemo, Yervoy increased median survival rates only somewhat. For a few lucky patients, however, the response to Yervoy was a dramatic improvement. Why some patients have responded better than others is still an unknown.

The "news" about lung cancer, in which I have a particular interest, was more muted. A small group of patients with small-cell lung cancer who also have the ALK gene mutation were treated with Pfizer's crizotinib. There appears to be some benefit from the drug, but there were no controlled study results that could be cited. It is somewhat disheartening that lung cancer is still not front and center.

The overall theme of this year's conference is the development of drug treatments based on individualized tumor biomarkers. Every day the biology of cancer is becoming better understood and that improved understanding is resulting in new breakthroughs in treatment. The breakthroughs and new treatments can't come fast enough.

It did not make the news, but I was astonished to learn that lung cancer is now the No. 1 killer in Charlotte County, surpassing heart disease, according to Virginia B Andes' Community Clinic Medical Director. Dr. Gonzales noted an increasing number of lung cancer cases presenting at our free clinic and did a little investigating. At a recent meeting of the clinic's board of directors he presented this startling statistic from the Health Planning Council of Southwest Florida.

The other interesting cancer-related news this week was about the World Health Organization's International Agency for Research on Cancer, coming out with the declaration that "radio frequency electromagnetic fields are possibly carcinogenic to humans, based on an increased risk of glioma, a malignant brain cancer."

The author of "The Secret History of the War on Cancer" and renowned epidemiologist, Dr. Devra Davis, testified before Congress about this issue not too long ago. Davis is said to have been initially a skeptic about cell phones being carcinogenic, but as she looked into the matter she found evidence showing how radio frequency could indeed damage DNA and potentially contribute to brain tumors. She now calls the issue "the most important and unrecognized public health issue of our time." In fact Davis has a new book entitled "Disconnect" detailing what her research has found. Davis can't tell you that cell phones are dangerous, but she can't tell you that they are safe either.

This debate will go on until there is definitive proof, decades from now, perhaps in the form of an epidemic of brain tumors. Of course, industry will fight to disprove the link and murky the scientific waters, the same way big tobacco tried to disprove the link between smoking and lung cancer. All I can say is, yeah right! Put me on speaker phone!

Lung Cancer Blues

Last week I got the good news that my PET/CT results were negative and there was no evidence of disease. Thank you Lord!

You would think that kind of news would get me all pumped up and raring to get on with life, but I am still in a funk and having a hard time getting into gear. This bill of good health comes with a price.

I have a cough that just won't quit, both feet hurt from peripheral neuropathy, I have a big toe on my right foot that feels like it is broken at the joint, and now I have back pain in my spine that feels like it could be arthritis. On top of this I am constantly having muscle cramps and spasms. One night last week I got a cramp in my calf so bad it made me jump out of bed at four in the morning swearing like a drunken sailor. (Yoko thought I was having a bad dream and tried to tackle me as I leapt from bed! In retrospect the whole incident was kind of comical, but it wasn't funny as it was happening!)

I've decided that I need to take care of these issues or my quality of life is going to suffer. My foot problems and constant hacking are keeping me from doing more vigorous exercise. I've complained about the toe and neuropathy to my doctors. I had a blood test done to check my uric acid level. It was elevated, but not high enough to indicate gout. An X-ray of the toe did not show anything definitive either. I have an appointment with a podiatrist next week to see if there is something else we can do.

As far as the cough goes, I'm not sure what more can be done. I've been taking an expectorant that seems to help. The cough is the result of the radiation to my right lung, which has produced scarring and a constant tickle in my chest. Any exertion that causes me to breathe deep also causes me to cough, sometime uncontrollably.

I've tried drinking more water and eating more bananas to get rid of the cramps, but as I type this my hands are starting to cramp again. I've been told that drinking tonic water (which has quinine in it) will help.

I can live with a little neuropathy, a sore toe, a cough, and periodic cramping. More worrying to me is the back pain, which has only developed recently. The PET/CT scans don't show anything and my CEA level (a biomarker for cancer) is holding steady. To eliminate the possibility that cancer has metastasized to the spine, I underwent an MRI today, just to be sure. I should know the results later this week.

The spine is the most common area for development of metastatic disease. According to one article I found, spine metastases occur in about 70% of cancer patients, but only 10% of those patients who have spine mets have symptoms during their lifetime. I found both those statistics rather surprising.

According to the article, the symptoms of spinal mets at first commonly resemble arthritis or a mild back strain that can be easily treated with Tylenol or ibuprofen. The pain becomes more constant and severe over a matter or days or weeks. (This sounds like me. I did not have back pain a month ago.)

According to the same article, spine mets can result in weakness to your arms and legs that can progress to paralysis in a short period of time. It's not something you want to fool with!

I met with my oncologist last week and he does not think I have metastatic disease. He's probably right. Just the same he agreed we should do the MRI, and get the answer, one way or the other. Stay tuned.

Arriving at a Turning Point

This past week certainly turned out well. My PET/CT scan results show no evidence of disease and the MRI showed no cancer. It did show that my arthritis-like back pain may be coming from some minor degenerative disease. I'm going to see a spine specialist to find out what, if anything can be done.

I feel like I've reached some turning point and I have to decide what direction my life takes from here. I now think that I will be a long-term cancer survivor, so I have to turn to planning our life in the long term. I didn't expect to be here three years ago, so I have not thought very much about the future.

When I first started working, I had hoped to make enough money to retire by the time I was 45. Let's just say that didn't work out. Over the last dozen years I've worked to build my business and provide for my family. All three of my daughters have finished college and are employed. My oldest daughter, Paula, has a family of her own. The other two have serious boyfriends. More weddings may be on the horizon.

On Father's Day I spoke with all three of my girls and the theme of the conversations were strikingly similar: where do we go from here?

Daughter Jessica found a job in St. Petersburg working for a small business that provides administrative services to non-profits. She moved out of our house and into an apartment this past week and started her working career on Monday. Her boyfriend, Matt, is a third-year law student at FSU. Jessie's plan for the moment is to work and save some money. For the time being she plans to stay here in Florida.

Middle daughter, June, has lived in Honolulu since her graduation from The University of Florida. She's been there for about five years and she is starting to develop island fever. June wants to find a job in California to be near her boyfriend, Will, who lives in San Diego. June sent me her resume and asked me to critique it this past week. My advice was to add an objective and to emphasize what she has accomplished. She doesn't know yet what she wants to do with her life. That's ok, I told her, I'm 56 years old and neither do I!

My eldest daughter Paula and her husband, Brian, live in California with Maddox, our baby grandson. Paula has found her calling as a teacher and completed her master's in education this past December. She is the planner in the family and on Father's day she told me that she and Brian have a five-year plan to move back to Florida so they can be closer to us. Wouldn't that be nice! Having the girls living here in Florida would take some of the uncertainty out of our plans for the future. Let's hope it happens. I'd like to be able to see my grandchildren more than once a year!

I figure I have about ten years left to before I can consider retiring. These last 10 years of my working life need to be my most productive. I've been thinking about what my ten year goals should be and the things I want to accomplish. Where do I want to be and what do I want to be doing? The possibilities abound.

Financial matters are on my mind of late. I want to be debt free with plenty of cash in the bank when I retire. Now that the kids are out of the house and on their own, I should be able to devote more resources toward securing our retirement future. I can only pray there are no more bumps in the road and everything from here out goes smoothly.

Southwest Florida Free to Breathe Event

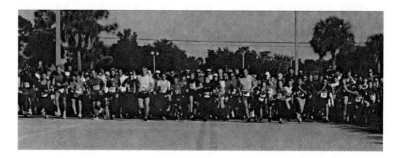

Photo Courtesy of Sun Newspapers

This October will mark four years since I was diagnosed with lung cancer. It is hard to believe that so much time has elapsed. I feel like I have accomplished so little in four years, especially when it comes to helping fund lung cancer research and awareness.

What motivated me to do something were the facts about where government spends the available cancer research dollars. There is no question that there is a direct correlation between research dollars invested and long term disease survival.

The best example is HIV/AIDS. The US government spends $3 billion on funding AIDS research annually, with the result that this dreaded disease, which was once highly stigmatized and nearly an immediate death sentence, now has a 90 percent three-year survival rate. The breakthrough was anti-retroviral drug therapy.

AIDS use to be seen as a "lifestyle" disease primarily affecting homosexuals and drug addicts. It was not until the people marched on Washington and demanded action that HIV/AIDS became a national research priority. Lung cancer, in similar fashion, is seen as a smoker's disease, even though most lung cancer patients today either quit smoking or never smoked. Millions of Americans are at risk of contracting and dying from lung cancer. It is hard for me to understand why so little is being done.

Despite the fact that lung cancer is the No. 1 cancer killer, the US government funding of lung cancer research is only $267 million. Private research funding is a mere $3 million annually. As a result the five-year survival rate for lung cancer has hardly changed in 30 years. It was 12 percent in the 1970s and today it is only 16 percent.

These facts led me to launch a personal crusade to do something about raising awareness and funding for lung cancer research. It did not take me long to realize that, without grassroots support, lobbying would be akin to howling at the moon. The key to success is widespread support.

What is needed is an organization focused on making lung cancer a national priority by building a grassroots effort and national support for change. The National Lung Cancer Partnership, founded by physicians and researchers, is the only national advocacy organization working with survivors and advocates, to decrease deaths due to lung cancer and help patients live longer and better through research and advocacy. In the past five years the partnership has funded $2 million in lung cancer research through the "Free to Breathe" event series. That's not a lot of money in the scheme of things, which gives rise to my frustration that we haven't been able to do more.

I organized the first "Free to Breathe" 5K Run/Walk in Southwest Florida in 2009 with some moderate success. We had more than 300 participants and raised about $30,000. That first year we only had four lung cancer survivors in attendance.

In 2010 our race gained about 25 percent more participants and nearly doubled our fundraising to about $54,000. Most important, we doubled the number of participating survivors.

Our goal for this year's event is to raise $100,000 and enroll 800 participants to run or walk.

Inspired By Inspire.com

When I was first diagnosed with cancer, I tried to get all the information I could about my disease. Naturally I used free online resources like The American Cancer Society's website (www.cancer.org). The ACS website provided me with basic authoritative information about my diagnosis (Stage IIIA adenocarcinoma) and treatment options. Today the ACS website even has an online "treatment wizard" that serves as a general clinical guide (not to be used as a substitute for a doctor), but there is a lot that the ACS "treatment wizard" leaves wanting.

The most burning question people with a devastating cancer diagnosis have is "What comes next?" A cancer diagnosis puts your life on hold until you have the answer to that question. And everyone is different. No one can tell you whether or not you will survive, how severe side effects from treatment may be, or what you can do about the unexpected side effects that frequently occur. They might tell you on the ACS website that a drug like Tarceva may cause a rash, but they don't necessarily tell you how best to treat it.

Four years ago I found an online website called www.inspire.com which brings together communities of people who either have a disease in common or is caring for someone. The communities of patients and caregivers on Inspire now total more than 300,000 at any given time. Categories of health topics and discussions groups range from autism, breast cancer and Alzheimer's to psoriasis, preemies, and women's heart disease. The website has blogs, journals, and discussion groups and is organized in a way that makes becoming involved easy and anonymous, if you so choose.

Once you become a member (registration is FREE and intrusive personal questions are minimal) you can elect to have a daily e-mail sent to you listing discussion topics that may be of interest. I'm a member of the online lung cancer support group, which, sadly, has 17,000 members and a load of new postings every day. If you post your own question or comment on the site you're sure to have multiple responses within hours.

Postings and discussions on Inspire cover such desperate issues as disability insurance and financial hardship, strains in relationships with people (family and friends) who "just can't deal" with cancer, the emotional toll of treatments on both patients and caregivers, and coping with end-stage disease and the loss of a loved one.

The website is called "Inspire" because the concept is for patients and survivors to give each other hope and inspiration as they battle their disease. It's a place to gain understanding from others who have been there and can share their experience and advice for any given situation. Every patient wants to know they can wake-up from their personal nightmare to a better day.

Among the more memorable recent postings, drawing hundreds of sympathetic responses was the story of a woman who complained her husband lost his job (and insurance coverage) because she had been diagnosed with lung cancer. Apparently, the employer decided to dismiss her husband, an 11-year veteran salesman in a small business, because he would have to be absent from work in order to care for his wife. It is hard to believe that anyone could be so heartless.

When I was in treatment, I remember asking about people's experience with shingles. At the time I did not know that chemo could weaken your immune system to the point where the chicken pox virus can potentially wreak painful havoc on your nervous system.

I also remember asking about what people had experienced with PCI (prophylactic cranial irradiation or whole brain radiation). My question ignited a firestorm of debate about the pros and cons of this controversial treatment option.

I ultimately decided to go ahead with PCI, and, so far, I am glad I did.

Sniffer Dogs Detect Lung Cancer

It is not often than lung cancer research makes the national news but this past week was an exception. An amazing breakthrough discovery was made. Trained dogs are able to detect lung cancer with uncanny accuracy. The story was covered on NBC Nightly News with Brian Williams and other national news outlets.

According to Science News, the study was carried out by Schillerhoehe Hospital in Germany. Lung cancer is the most common cause of death from cancer worldwide. It kills 340,000 men and women in Europe and 160,000 Americans each year.

Lung cancer has high mortality because there is no reliable method for early detection and patients show no outward symptoms until the disease has irreversibly progressed. Methods for screening and early detection would significantly improve survival and reduce mortality.

Scientists theorize that identifying VOC (volatile organic compounds) linked to the presence of cancer could be a key to early detection. The new study aimed at finding out if trained sniffer dogs could be used to detect lung cancer on the breath of lung cancer patients. A dog's sense of smell is much more sensitive than humans. A dog has 220 million olfactory receptors in its nose, compared with just five million for humans.

The study included 220 volunteers with COPD, lung cancer patients, and a cohort of healthy people. The trained dogs in the study correctly identified 71 samples with lung cancer out of a possible 100. They also correctly detected 372 samples that did not have lung cancer out of a possible 400.

The dogs could detect lung cancer independently from COPD and tobacco smoke. What is exciting is that these results confirm the presence of a stable marker for lung cancer that is independent of COPD and also detectable in the presence of tobacco smoke, food odors and drugs.

The next step will be to identify those specific compounds observed in the exhaled breath of patients. There is still quite a bit of detective work left to be done, but at least we know we're on the right track! Way to go Fido!

There was other news this week regarding lung cancer research that got my attention.

I've always wondered why some people (smokers and non-smokers) develop lung cancer while others do not. Only 15 percent of all smokers develop lung cancer, so it stands to reason that there must be some difference between those smokers and non-smokers who develop the disease and the vast majority of people who do not.

According to online resource Science Daily, scientists have now discovered that smokers with variations in two specific genes have a greater risk of smoking more cigarettes, becoming more dependent on nicotine and developing lung cancer.

The scientific community is increasingly focusing research efforts on finding genetic differences between different cohorts of people. This kind of effort may eventually lead to a genetic test to identify people at higher risk for developing lung cancer.

I also learned this week that a series of studies funded by the National Lung Cancer Partnership have resulted in promising new developments for the treatment of lung cancer.

Drs. Richard Pietras and Lee Goodglick from the Geffen School of Medicine at UCLA and the Jonsson Comprehensive Cancer Center discovered that estrogen drives the growth of many non-small cell lung cancers (NSCLC). Lung tumors create aromatase, the enzyme responsible for a key step in estrogen synthesis.

A laboratory experiment treating NSCLC with a common chemotherapy drug, Cisplatin, showed only a modest and temporary effect on the tumor. However, when Cisplatin was combined with aromatase inhibitors (drugs used to stop the production of estrogen — the same ones used to treat breast cancer), the combination appeared to completely eliminate the tumor.

These studies also suggest that the effects of this interaction can reverse tumor resistance to Cisplatin. The drugs being tested are already FDA-approved. The next step is a clinical trial.

Is Whole Brain Radiation a Good Idea?

The issue of whether or not to have whole brain radiation keeps coming up as a contentious issue within our online lung cancer support group. I have had an opportunity to weigh in on the issue numerous times, but I thought it would be good to summarize my position and how I came to a decision about this treatment option.

I finished chemo on May 30 2008. At that point my oncologist told me that there was nothing further to do, other than perhaps WBR (whole brain radiation). (When you do WRB without having any detectable tumors, it is known as PCI — Prophylactic Cranial Irradiation). The idea is to irradiate the brain before the cancer can metastasize to the brain.

My understanding is that the more robust the response lung cancer patients have to chemo and radiation, the more likely it is that the cancer will move to the brain. The way I think of it like a round-up. We poisoned the body and killed most of the cancer — to the point where it is not now detectable. The only place of "escape" is the brain, where the blood-brain barrier prevents chemo from working effectively on cancerous cells. PCI will (theoretically) take care of any cancer cells hiding in the brain.

Knowing that after consolidation chemo there is no further treatment that we can PROACTIVELY do, I considered whether or not going the next step to PCI was worth the risk. I asked the question to my online lung cancer support group. To say the least, the responses were not encouraging. Here is one reply regarding side effects:

Radiation Therapy Side Effects

The side effects of Radiation Therapy can be classified as acute, sub-acute and delayed. Acute reactions occur during the course of treatment and are temporary. They are manifested as signs of increased inter-cranial pressure or worsening of neurological deficits. They result from an increase in cerebral edema (abnormal accumulation of fluid). The administration of corticosteroids usually decreases or alleviates symptoms. Steroids are generally administered during the course of therapy to prevent this occurrence. Other acute reactions are nausea, vomiting, anorexia (loss of appetite), fatigue, alopecia (loss of hair) and skin irritation.

Delayed reactions usually occur 6-24 months after completion of therapy. These effects are irreversible and often progressive. They result from direct injury to brain tissue and blood vessels. These reactions are due to changes in the white matter and death of brain tissue caused by radiation-damaged blood vessels. Symptoms vary from mild to severe decreased intellect, memory impairment, confusion, personality changes and alteration of the normal function of the area irradiated.

Long-term effects can be initially managed to some degree with corticosteroids and surgery to remove necrotic tissue. Other long-term reactions include loss of vision, development of secondary malignancies (oncogenesis) and pituitary-hypothalamic dysfunction (changes in normal hormone levels) leading to problems with your thyroid, sugar metabolism, fertility or ability to process water.

Sources: International Journal of Radiation Oncology, University of Pittsburgh Medical Center

You get the idea. Electing to have PCI was not something you decide lightly. I spoke at length with my doctors, other cancer patients, and researched what I could on the Internet. At the end of the day, there were no medical studies that said it was PROVEN to be a good idea, but then, there were no studies that said it was NOT! Part of the problem here is that your doctor does not want to give medical advice that is not "evidenced based." The fact of the matter is, while it might make logical sense, it has not been proven and is therefore not typically recommended.

I decided that I would rather be dummied down by brain radiation than dead. What do I have to lose? If I don't do it and develop brain cancer, I will kick myself for not having tried. If I never develop brain cancer I will look back on it as having perhaps been a contributor to helping me survive. If I get brain cancer three years from now, who is to say I would not have developed it anyway? The way I looked at it, I have little to lose and everything to gain by giving it a try.

Once the set-up was complete, I went to the radiologist every day before work for three weeks, with each session lasting only a few minutes (2 grays per day X 15 days). The 30 grays were half of what I got in radiation to my right lung. I was lucky in that I was able to complete the treatment without the use of steroids. The only side effect was the loss of hair. I was losing it in patches and decided to simply shave my head.

I am glad to have done this as I don't believe I am going to suffer any bad side effects. I want to have done everything possible to prevent the cancer from returning.

Realistically I know that the cancer can (and probably will) come back. I would like to at least have the satisfaction of having put up a good fight!

Indicator Lights Signal Trouble

My sister Jane and her husband David live at Smith Mountain Lake near Roanoke, Virginia. We had made plans a few months ago to get together at the lake towards the end of the summer. Yoko and I didn't really have plans to take a summer vacation this year, so visiting Jane and David was, for us, the next best thing.

Our plan was to take an early morning flight on Allegiant Air from St Pete to Roanoke on Friday, arriving in Roanoke at 9 AM. Rather than getting up in the middle of the night to go to St. Pete, we decided instead to drive up on Thursday evening and stay with my daughter, Jessie, who lives just 15 minutes from the airport. Of course, as is often the case, things did not go as planned.

My car, a small two-seater hard-top convertible, was acting up on Thursday. The "check engine" indicator light was on and I was afraid we might have trouble getting to St. Pete. When I got home from work, we decided to take Yoko's car, a large four door sedan, instead. It was raining at 5 PM when we left our home.

Traffic slowed as a car waited to make a left turn into a strip mall on the left. A white SUV in front of me slowed down and I, in turn, slowed almost to a complete stop when the car behind me slammed into the back of our car.

I stood on my brakes and just barely avoided hitting the car in front of me. The speed of the impact was such that, had we been in my little two-seater, we might have been severely injured. It was a good thing we were in the sedan. That "check engine" indicator light in the sports car may have saved us.

The car that hit me was driven by a 16 year-old girl, who, obviously, was not paying attention. Luckily, no one was badly injured. I hit the top of my head on the visor causing an abrasion and had some minor neck and shoulder pain. As a precaution, I decided to go to the hospital by ambulance to get checked out. Yoko said she was fine and declined treatment. It took about three and a half hours before I was released from the hospital with a clean bill of health. In the meantime, Yoko drove our damaged car home and came to the hospital in my small convertible.

We grabbed a bite to eat and headed to St. Pete, arriving at 10:30 PM. The check engine indicator light did NOT come on again the entire trip. It made me think that God most certainly was watching over us.

Friday morning we were up at 5:00 AM for our 7:30 AM flight to Virginia. The plane departed the gate on time but halfway down the runway, the pilot aborted the takeoff. Apparently the right engine indicator light had gone off, signaling trouble. We waited in the plane for about a half an hour while the mechanics looked to see what the problem might be. We tried taking off again about an hour later, but again half way down the runway, the pilot aborted takeoff for a second time!

I've flown all over the world in the past 40 years and I have never once been on an aborted takeoff. I was really beginning to think our quick trip to Virginia was not meant to be! After a few hours of waiting for a replacement plane, we were, at last, airborne.

We had a lot of fun visiting Jane and David and spending a few very special days with them. Thank God (or saints in heaven) for the check engine indicator lights that allowed us to arrive safely.

Survived by His Wife

A friend of mine sent me a funny YouTube video of an old nightclub routine done by the legendary comedian Allen King called "Survived by his Wife."

King's act was about how women tend to outlive their husbands. In the video, the comedian claims that he had to defend himself from women advocates who called him a "male chauvinist pig" after he remarked that women outlive men because "women don't have a wife." His routine revolves around having to "defend himself" by having randomly selected women in the audience verify and read actual newspaper obituaries.

No matter what the manner of death or how old or infirm the man might be, the deceased is always "survived by his wife." Like all comedy, the joke contains an element of truth, which is what makes it funny.

King's bit concludes with an obituary that reports of how a woman, learning that her husband was having an extramarital affair, decides to end it all by flinging herself from the roof of a three-story building. She survives the fatal fall by landing on her husband, killing him.

The truth is that women generally outlast their husbands, whatever the reason. But lung cancer in women is on the rise and is beginning to strike younger women — even children — with alarming frequency.

Case in point: Kara Kennedy, the daughter of the late Senator Ted Kennedy, was diagnosed with lung cancer in 2002, at the age of 42 at the time. She lived as a survivor and cancer free for six years. She died unexpectedly from heart failure this week at the age of 51. Was her heart failure somehow related to lung cancer treatments? No one knows for sure, but treatment for lung cancer may have played some role. Sadly, she is survived by her ex-husband and their two teenage children.

What triggered me to write about women and lung cancer this week was the generous and unsolicited donation I received from the Rotonda West Women's Club, which is headed by club president Doris Walker. I was invited by Doris to speak to the group this past January and made some emotional remarks about lung cancer and my personal campaign for funding and awareness.

I must have struck a chord. The club asked me back to speak at their September meeting and presented me with a generous $1,000 donation to the National Lung Cancer Partnership.

During the presentation, I asked the assembled women how many knew someone with lung cancer. A great many hands went up, including quite a number of women who related how they had lost their husband to lung cancer. It made me think that lung cancer victims are frequently "survived by their wife."

I spoke to the club about participating in the up-coming Free to Breathe event and why I think it is so important to raise awareness about lung cancer as well as funding for research. This group of ladies got the message. Not only did they present me with a giant check, they registered a large walking team at www.freetobreathe.com. The team is called the "Rotonda Walking Wonders", led by Rose Marie Morris. Their goal is to raise $1,500 for our event and I have no doubt they will succeed.

The Rotonda West Women's Club made me realize that I should try to get in front of other groups, especially women. When it comes to fundraising for cancer, or other important causes for that matter, women get things done.

Four Years and Counting

I was diagnosed with lung cancer exactly four-years ago this week. These days I consider October to be the anniversary of a second chance at life.

I'm a miracle boy, the rare four year survivor of Stage IIIA adenocarcinoma. I thank God for every new day. The silver lining of a cancer diagnosis is that you realize the importance of making each day count. Life is too short to waste.

I've been thinking about what I have been able to accomplish and experience in the past four years. How truly miraculous these years have been! First of all, I've had the time to see my youngest daughter, Jessica, graduate from college. My oldest daughter, Paula, is now married, earned a master's degree in education, and has become a mother. I hope I live long enough to walk my other daughters down the aisle.

Four years ago I realized that I might not be around to tell my life stories. I didn't want to die without leaving some sort of record, so I began writing. A year later my blog turned into a newspaper column, which I have written for one-hundred and sixty straight weeks. (Those columns turned into this book!)

At the time of my diagnosis I was helping launch the Virginia B. Andes Volunteer Community Clinic. While undergoing treatments, I served as treasurer of the organization. I worked to get the fledgling clinic and pharmacy funded and on a sound financial footing. I subsequently succeeded Dr. David Klein as president of the board. The Virginia B Andes free clinic has become an indispensable part of the social safety net in Charlotte County and I am very proud to have played a role in its founding. Other than raising my daughters, nothing I have done in my life has been more satisfying.

I got involved with advocating for the National Lung Cancer Partnership after I learned about the lack of funding for lung cancer research. I was stunned to learn that lung cancer, the number one cancer killer, receives less federal research funding than any other cancer group. That is inexplicable to me and needs to change.

For the past three years I've been on a crusade to raise awareness and funding for lung cancer research. I organized the SW Florida Free to Breathe 5K Run/Walk in 2009 and 2010, which together raised $84,000. This year the goal is to raise $100,000 and have 800 participants.

I have a full time job and have worked hard to build my business. It hasn't been easy, especially in the current economic environment. With the help of my partner we've managed to double revenues these past four years, which thankfully provides us with a modicum of financial stability. I am blessed to have a great partner and wonderful clients who have stuck with us through thick and thin.

I continue to be an active member of the Harbor Heights Peace River Rotary, a great way to give back to the community, network, and make a positive contribution. The men in this club are my brothers.

Were it not for Rotary, I might never have gone to Japan, met my wife or have the life I am living today. Rotary's motto is "Service

Above Self," which, I now know, is also profound advice for a happy and fulfilling life.

A Tribute to Steve Jobs

Steve Jobs, the co-founder of Apple, died this week after a heroic battle with pancreatic cancer. His death certificate said he died of "respiratory arrest," a result of metastatic disease.

Steve knew he was dying seven years ago, when he was first diagnosed. I think people will say that these past seven years were the most productive of his life.

Steve and I were both born in 1955. I have always felt some special connection to him, even though I never even met the man. He was a famous, multimillionaire 20-year-old I read about in magazines when I was an anonymous college student without a penny to my name. Steve was changing the world with his revolutionary personal computer and graphical user interface. He was making the cover of Time while I was struggling just to support myself. By his many achievements, Steve Jobs made a whole generation of Americans feel inadequate.

In all honesty, I admired Steve Jobs. He was the kind of person I wanted to be. I am sad that he is gone. I feel like I have lost a close friend.

Steve and I grew up together. We were teenagers in the 1960's. We were both in second grade when Kennedy was shot. We listened to the same music, read the same books and magazines, and experienced a rapidly changing world in the same way. Steve and I had the same opportunities in life, but look at what he was able to accomplish with his 56 years. Imagine what he might have accomplished if he had lived another two decades.

I've been reading a lot about Steve Jobs' life in the past week and I continue to be amazed by all that he accomplished. I read the commencement address he made at Stanford, after he had been diagnosed with cancer, and I was struck by how much I could relate to what he was saying.

One passage was particularly insightful into the mind of someone living with cancer:

"Remembering that I'll be dead soon is the most important tool I've ever encountered to help me make the big choices in life. Because almost everything — all external expectations, all pride, all fear of embarrassment or failure — these things just fall away in the face of death, leaving only what is truly important. Remembering that you are going to die is the best way I know to avoid the trap of thinking you have something to lose. You are already naked. There is no reason not to follow your heart."

Those are words a cancer survivor can understand in a way that few of the young graduates at Stanford could. One thing I know is that Steve Jobs has taught us all to live every day as if it were your last and to follow your dreams, wherever they may take you.

Job's gave his commencement speech at Stanford in 2005. At the time he thought his cancer had been cured with surgery and his medical trauma had ended with the procedure he had endured. He said:" This was the closest I've been to facing death, and I hope it's the closest I get for a few more decades. Having lived through it, I can now say this to you with a bit more certainty than when death was a useful but purely intellectual concept: No one wants to die. Even people who want to go to heaven don't want to die to get there. And yet death is the destination we all share. No one has ever escaped it. And that is as it should be, because Death is very likely the single best invention of Life. It is Life's change agent. It clears out the old to make way for the new. Right now the new is you, but someday not too long from now, you will gradually become the old and be cleared away."

Well said! Steve Jobs was a hero to me and his own generation. He will be sorely missed and long remembered.

The Spin Doctors

One of my favorite jokes from the early 1980's goes like this:

God appeared to U.S. President Ronald Reagan, Soviet Premier Mikhail Gorbachev, and Prime Minister of Israel Yitzhak Shamir, telling them that they must warn their people that He plans to destroy the world in three days.

President Reagan appears on national TV and says, "My fellow Americans, I have good news and bad news. The good news is there is a God. The bad news is He will destroy the world in three days."

Premier Gorbachev goes on Soviet television and announces "Comrades, I have bad news and worse news. The bad news is there is a God. The worse news is He plans to destroy the world in three days."

Finally, Prime Minister Shamir addresses the people of Israel, saying, "Good people of Israel, I have wonderful news and better news! The wonderful news is that there is a God! The better news is that there will never be a Palestinian state!"

I always thought that story was funny as a commentary on how politicians "spin" the facts, depending on who is telling the story. What I never realized was how blind we are to reality!

I've been reading a fascinating book by famed psychologist Daniel Kahneman called "Thinking, Fast and Slow." The book is about how the human mind works and flaws in human decision making. I picked the book up to gain a better understanding of my own decision making mechanisms and biases. But I am also discovering how easily the mind can be tricked and made to believe things that are not true.

The book caught my attention because it argues that people frequently don't make rational economic choices, which flies in the face of conventional wisdom. As a financial advisor, I thought this would be important information to know.

As someone who never took a course in psychology, even the elementary examples of how the mind can be tricked are fascinating. One example is to ask someone how many animals of each kind Moses took into the ark.

As your mind races to answer the question, it may never occur to you the answer is zero. Noah gathered the animals, not Moses! For most people it doesn't even register that the question was about Moses, not Noah.

Kahneman offers the hypothesis that the mind is composed of two systems, which he calls System One (fast thinking) and System Two (slow thinking). To demonstrate the workings of fast thinking, he shows a picture of an angry woman. You instantly and effortlessly recognize the woman's facial features as that of anger. He then asks you to solve 17 X 24 in your head. Coming to an answer takes some effort and concentration (slow thinking) before you recognize the correct answer, which is 408. What the book is about is the relationship and interaction between these two systems.

So what does a book on psychology have to do with living with cancer? Actually, quite a lot, especially when we are talking about the relationship between fast and slow thinking and human perception and decision making. The book is filled with cancer examples and common misperceptions by both patients and doctors alike.

It occurs to me that people have the widespread belief that breast cancer is a more prevalent and deadlier form of cancer than it actually is. Kahneman's book provides an explanation for such misperceptions with what he calls the availability heuristic.

The basic idea of the availability heuristic is that the more frequently you hear about something, the more easily instances can be recalled. The more easily something is recalled, the more likely it is to be judged "large" by the fast system.

After reading this book I realized how easily our minds can be persuaded that something false is true and visa versa. No wonder we have the expression "spin doctors" for people who try to get into our head to influence our decisions. It's easier than I would ever have imagined.

Discovering Eva Cassidy

The Internet and a variety of new electronic devices make accessing and listening to the kind of music I love easy. I use Pandora on my iPad to stream the music of my favorite artists. Bluegrass legend Allison Krause is among my favorites.

Listening to the Allison Krause music "station" on Pandora the other day I discovered an artist named Eva Cassidy. Her music was so stunningly beautiful that I immediately decided to purchase her best-selling album, "Songbird." I was mesmerized by the voice of this woman. How could it be that I had never heard of Eva Cassidy until now?

I went to YouTube to see if I could find videos of her performing. What I found was an ABC news report about the life of Eva Cassidy and her rise to fame. Eva never enjoyed celebrity while she was alive. She played local clubs in the Washington D.C. area and lived by selling CDs out of the trunk of her car. She died in obscurity in 1996.

According to Wikipedia, Cassidy's music was first brought to the attention of British audiences when her version of "Over the Rainbow" was played on BBC Radio. Following an overwhelming response to the broadcast, a home made video recording of "Over the Rainbow" was shown on BBC's Top of the Pops 2. That recording, taken with a camcorder at Blues Alley in Washington D.C., is on YouTube for posterity.

If you have never heard Eva Cassidy sing, you simply must.

How good was Eva Cassidy? In 2005 Amazon.com released a list of its top 25 best-selling musicians. Cassidy placed fifth, behind the likes of The Beatles, U2, and Norah Jones and far ahead of Elvis Presley and many other well-known stars. Her Songbird album sold millions of copies after her death. Imagine the career she might have had were she alive today! One famed music critic acclaims Eva Cassidy as one of the greatest singers of our generation. I am not sure which is more tragic; her premature death or the fact that she never achieved fame while she was alive.

Cassidy had a malignant mole removed from her back in 1993. Three years later, during a promotional event for the Live at Blues Alley album in July 1996, she noticed an ache in her hips. The pain persisted and a few weeks later, X-rays revealed that the melanoma had spread to her lungs and bones. She died of cancer at her family home in Bowie, Maryland on November 2, 1996, at the age of 33.

Cancer not only takes the life of its victim. It robs all of us of a precious life from whom we might all benefit. No one is more devastated by cancer than the patient, but we all lose when someone so young and full of promise dies.

In the case of Eva Cassidy clearly what we lost was an extraordinary musical talent and an opportunity to have had a large body of work and a lifetime full of achievement. Eva refused to be pigeonholed into one genre. She sang jazz, country, blues, traditional and gospel like nobody else.

Instead of having a vast repertoire, we are left with just two CD recordings, some videos, and dreams of what might have been. Eva Cassidy was cheated out of life at a young age and I feel cheated not to have known her while she was alive and not to be able to look forward to her next album.

Like many musicians, Eva Cassidy had no insurance. She neglected to do proper surveillance after having that malignant mole removed from her back. Undoubtedly, lack of insurance resulted in her deciding to not to have regular doctor visits, which ultimately lead to her death. She died from metastatic cancer to her lung and bones. What a shame and what a waste.

Pizza as a Vegetable

I am pretty upset with our government and the way things get done in Washington. The latest news item to earn my ire was last week's "60 Minutes" story about how Congress is exempt from insider trading laws. People in political office are becoming wealthy as a result of their public service. If we as ordinary citizens were to trade on insider information, we'd go to jail. Exempting Congress is not right, but that's just the latest example of how our government representatives put themselves ahead of the American people.

Congressional approval is at an all-time low — just 9 percent — for good reason. Last week, in the debate over how to reduce childhood obesity, Congress effectively declared pizza to be a vegetable. Actually, what they did was to make it easier for the amount of tomato sauce that is on a pizza to satisfy school lunch nutritional regulations. The end result is the same. Pizza, by congressional action, now satisfies the vegetable requirement for school lunches. You've got to be kidding me. Simple common sense once again gives way to special interests and legal hair splitting.

I just finished reviewing scientific grant proposals for the government-funded Cancer Prevention Research Institute of Texas. Several proposals I read suggested targeting childhood obesity as a cancer preventative since we know that cancer and obesity are closely related in adulthood. One idea was to teach inner-city kids about good nutrition by having them plant vegetable gardens and learn to grow the food they consume at lunchtime. These are kids who become obese because they know nothing about good nutrition and healthy eating. There is no one at home to teach them.

But why even bother having a program to teach good nutrition if the government itself is just going to undermine the effort? If Congress can't agree that banning pizza and soft drinks from school lunches is a good idea as a first step toward dealing with childhood obesity, how on earth are they going to tackle the even more pressing and controversial issues facing our nation?

The fact of the matter is that our national debt is tied directly to our nation's health. If we ever want to do something about getting skyrocketing medical costs under control, we need to do something about the root causes to our poor health as a nation, including common addictions, a generally poor diet and lack of exercise in our daily life. What could be more important?

Imagine how much money we could save if government focused on drug and alcohol addiction, reducing obesity and promoting wellness. It would be transformative to our physical and financial health. We need political leadership to get there.

The truth is that government helped to create the lung cancer epidemic we have today. Generations of Americans have been addicted to nicotine thanks to the misguided notion that cigarettes in GI mess kits would be a good idea. (I would not be at all surprised to learn that big tobacco lobbied Congress to get cigarettes into mess kits, just as the frozen pizza industry lobbied to get pizza into school lunch programs.) What is good for public health was not a consideration.

The consequences of smoking only came to light years after GIs returned home addicted to nicotine. According to various Internet sources, smoking in the U.S. jumped 75 percent from 1940 to 1945 with the average annual consumption hitting a heart-stopping 3,500 cigarettes per person.

Cigarette addiction is one of the major reasons that heart disease and lung cancer are today the two leading causes of death in the United States. We can put the blame squarely on the shoulders of government.

Childhood obesity in America is a similar slow moving train wreck. Significantly higher rates of diabetes and cancer are on the horizon if we don't get the obesity problem under control. Banning pizza and soft drinks from school lunches would be a good start.

The Business of Cancer

I was scheduled to have a PET/CT examine as part of the surveillance program to monitor me for a recurrence of lung cancer. I have been having these tests every six months for the past four years. I don't mind the CT scan, which is like an X-ray in slices. You're in and out in no time. I don't like taking the more elaborate PET scan but I suffer through it because early detection is the one thing that could save my life.

I was surprised today when the imaging technician told me we would only be doing a CT scan. I had mentally steeled myself to take the PET and had anticipated both scans taking most of the morning. Apparently, my doctor's orders were over-ridden by my insurance company, Cigna, which only agreed to cover the less expensive CT.

I did not have a chance to speak with my oncologist, but obviously if he ordered a PET/CT, those are the surveillance tests he would prefer to see. I was somewhat irked that the insurance company would not authorize the PET scan, so I called Cigna to get an explanation.

I was told Cigna only discusses coverage decisions with healthcare providers, not patients! That doesn't seem right since I am the one paying the premiums, but I can understand their reasoning. (As a layman, they presume I am not in a position to understand or argue clinical decisions.)

When I got home I had a letter explaining how the decision to deny PET scan coverage was made and what the procedure is to appeal this decision.

To avoid the appearance of a conflict of interest, Cigna delegates coverage decisions regarding imaging diagnostics to a company named Med Solutions, an independent contractor. That seems fine on the surface, I suppose. My only question is what is the financial relationship between Cigna and Med Solutions? How does Med Solutions bill Cigna for its services? (Not surprisingly, that information was not disclosed in the documents I received.)

After the CT was done I went to get my blood drawn at the cancer clinic. As was the case at the imaging center, I drove around a jam-packed parking lot, unable to find space for my little car. Every car in the lot represented someone battling cancer. Sadly, in the midst of a recession, it's a booming business in Florida.

My experience this week served to remind me that, while I consider cancer to be a life-threatening disease, to radiologists, oncologists, hospitals, insurance companies, pharmaceutical companies etc., it's a business. And like all businesses, there is a need to grow and be profitable. I get it and I don't have a problem with the business of cancer per se, so long as the incentives are designed, first and foremost, to save or extend the patient's life. I certainly would not want to risk my life to save the insurance company money.

Just how big is the cancer business? According to the American Cancer Society, the annual cost of cancer in 2010 was $263 billion dollars, including $103 billion in direct medical costs. (Indirect costs, from loss of productivity due to illness or premature death are estimated at another $160 billion a year.)

The National Cancer Institute estimates that the medical cost of cancer in 2020 will grow to $158 billion to $178 billion, due to an aging population and other factors.

That's a big market by any measure. How on earth will we ever keep greed at bay?

It's a Wonderful Life

One my favorite movies is the Frank Capra Christmas classic *It's A Wonderful Life* starring Jimmy Stewart and Donna Reed. I love this movie for many reasons.

First of all, it is primarily a story about self-sacrifice, which is the central calling of Christianity — to sacrifice your own life for the sake of others. It's also a story about love, family, loyalty, heroism, trust, integrity, and generosity.

George Bailey, the main character, dreams about leading an adventurous life and traveling the world. Circumstances and the needs of family continually intervene to prevent him from ever leaving the fictional New York town of Bedford Falls.

George is portrayed as an everyday hero who quietly changes people's lives. He has a bad ear, so he can't serve in the military when war comes along. Ironically, his bad ear is the result of jumping into freezing water to save his brother's life. But it is his brother who becomes the war hero, not George.

At the end of the movie George becomes so despondent about his hum-drum life that he considers killing himself by jumping off a bridge. God sends Clarence, an angel, to save George Bailey and to reveal the meaning of his life — what the town of Bedford Falls would be like had he never been born. George comes to realize that the things he did with his life has had a profound effect on his community and the world.

The final scene in the movie is the outpouring of generosity when the town thinks that George himself could be in trouble.

What made me think of this movie? This past weekend we held the Third Annual Free to Breathe 5K Run/Walk and One Mile Memorial walk at Charlotte Sports Park to raise money for the National Lung Cancer Partnership and lung cancer research. I felt like George Bailey with all my friends and neighbors rushing to aid me in my hour of need.

I started the Southwest Florida Free to Breathe together with Florida Cancer Specialists in 2009. The first year of the race we had 300 participants and raised about $30,000. In 2010 the race grew to 400 participants and we raised $54,000, including a generous $10,000 post-event donation from the South Florida Ford Dealers. This year the race nearly doubled in size to 800 participants. We were able to raise $78,000, including $38,000 in corporate sponsorships and roughly $40,000 in registration fees and donations.

The SW Florida Free to Breathe event was our first opportunity to announce the formation of the Florida Chapter of the National Lung Cancer Partnership. Going forward, 25 percent of everything we raise in the State of Florida will be used locally in support of our mission to raise awareness and funding for lung cancer research. I will be serving as the Chapter's first president.

One famous line in "It's a Wonderful Life" is, "no man is poor who has friends." I feel very rich indeed to have so many friends and supporters. Thank you all!

Putting the Pieces Together

Have you ever watched a movie that has things happening and as you watch, you don't really understand what is happening or why?

I recently watched *Edge of Darkness* in which Mel Gibson, playing the part of a detective, uncovers a conspiracy following the grisly murder of his political-activist daughter. The movie's plot comes together like pieces of a puzzle to get to the heart of why his daughter was killed. In the end it all made sense, but at the start you are baffled about what is happening on screen and why.

Leonardo DiCaprio's *Shutter Island* or George Clooney's movie *Michael Clayton* are other examples of clarity coming at the end of the story. It occurs to me that life in general is a puzzle that requires you putting the pieces together to make sense. It is only by living that you begin to understand life and the world in which we live. The meaning of life comes at the end, like the conclusion of a movie such as *Mr. Holland's Opus*.

Things happen in life and you wonder what the import could be. What are we supposed to do with the gift of life that has been given to us? Is it all about surviving and fighting to meet our everyday needs? Or is there something else? Is there a higher purpose? God has a plan for all of us, but it is up to us to find out what it may be.

I've had occasion to think about this a lot since I was diagnosed with cancer. My career has taken me all over the world and given me something of a broad prospective about people, cultures, and life in general. One thing that I learned from all my travels is that the needs and desires of people all over the world are the same — to live and be happy. That means having food, clothing and shelter and to love and be loved. The sad truth is that most people who share our world don't have enough to eat or wear, or even a comfortable place to sleep.

This week the CBS news magazine "60 Minutes" featured a story about a 77-year-old man named Eli Broad whose goal in life is to give away the billions he earned as co-founder of KB Homes and later the owner of insurance giant Sun America. Broad purchased the family-owned insurer to diversify out of the cyclical home building business. He paid $52 million for Sun America in 1971 and sold it to AIG for $18 billion dollars in 1999.

Broad's philanthropic interests include education, science and the arts and he has already given away more than $2 billion in support of his favorite charities. It occurred to me that Eli Broad, now nearing the end of his life, wants to continue to live through his good works. The story of Broad's philanthropy reminds me of the Egyptians pharaohs creating monuments to mark their lives. We all can't be philanthropists on the gigantic scale of Eli Broad, but that does not diminish our natural human desire to be remembered or to do something good.

I thought it ironic that the story that followed on "60 Minutes" was about the monastic life of devoted Greek Orthodox monks who have no worldly ambitions. Their goal in life is to prepare for the hereafter. It struck me that Eli Broad's goal isn't much different, he's just gone about it in another way.

Life is a puzzle offering each of us different paths to happiness and salvation. Yoko and I are reaching the culmination of our life together. Our youngest daughter, Jessica, graduates this weekend from Florida State and in May Yoko and I will celebrate 30 years of marriage. The next stage of our life offers many possibilities and opportunities to make a contribution and a difference.

What Makes a Hero?

I have never done anything heroic. I was born 10 years after the end of World War II. I came of age during the Vietnam War era. Most of the people I knew in high school were looking for ways to avoid the draft. Only a few joined the military voluntarily. By the time I was college age the draft had ended. I applied to attend West Point, where my uncle was teaching, but failed to get an appointment. I often wonder what my life would be like today had I received that appointment and entered the military.

My uncle, Col. Timothy H. Donovan, was awarded (among many other commendations) the Silver Star for heroism in Vietnam during his second tour of duty. I was looking for the citation on the Internet and found an interview about what happened on November 1 1969, the day he was wounded.

First Platoon of Charlie Troop, 10th Cavalry, 4th Infantry Division, was ambushed by North Vietnamese forces. Charlie Troop's Commander was my uncle, Captain Timothy H. Donovan. According to the article, he "instinctively ordered his remaining soldiers to counterattack and simultaneously maneuvered his headquarters element into the heart of the action. As the battle unfolded, a North Vietnamese sniper (waiting patiently in a "spider hole") managed to squeeze off a round from his AK-47 that would forever change the face of the United States Military."

The interview goes on to explain that "the sniper's bullet entered through the seam of his flak jacket, broke several ribs, burst his left lung, and pierced his pulmonary artery before riddling its way down his spinal column and lodging itself in his spleen.

A few hours later, an Army surgeon stood over a bloody M.A.S.H. operating table and declared that it was "too late for this one." His plans changed when Donovan (with two collapsed lungs) reached up and grabbed him by the throat with his right hand. In that instance, the fate of countless service men and women changed forever."

My uncle continued serving in the military even though he was wheelchair bound that first year. He learned to walk with crutches, then two canes, and then one. He went on to have a brilliant military career lasting more than two decades.

Among his assignments, he was deeply involved with planning for desert warfare at the Pentagon. He taught tactics and military history at West Point and apparently had students named Petraeus and McCrystal. He was in charge of taking Special Operations Command from concept to reality during the Reagan era. He became the commanding officer of a regiment in Germany responsible for the deployment of tanks to NATO. In fact, one was issued to his son, Mike, who fought with it in Desert Storm. My uncle retired from the military a full colonel. Today he lives a quiet, unassuming life in Virginia.

All week I have been watching the pictures coming out of Japan and I have been thinking about what makes a hero. I've come to the conclusion that heroes are people who knowingly put themselves in harm's way for the sake of others. Our men and women in uniform certainly fit the bill. So do the plant workers at Fukushima who are subjecting themselves to radiation exposure that is likely to destroy their health, if not take their life. I can't say how much I admire these people and the selfless sacrifice they are making.

I was thinking of flying to Japan and volunteering to help, but I am afraid I'd just get in the way. Still, it's frustrating to watch the news, day after day, and feel powerless to make a difference.

It's the same feeling I have when I am approached by someone with cancer wanting to know what can be done. I wish there was more I could do.

Why I Advocate for Lung Cancer

Let's get this out of the way first, because it is the first question people ask when I tell them I have lung cancer.

Yes, I was a cigarette smoker. I picked up the smoking habit when I was a 17-year old high school exchange student living in Osaka, Japan. It was 1972 and everyone in Japan smoked. I took up cigarettes just to fit in. By the time I was 20 I was ready to quit. The problem was by then I was addicted. It took me 35 years to finally kick the habit. I tried and failed many times. I finally succeeded the year before I was diagnosed with locally advanced Stage IIIA adenocarcinoma (non-small cell lung cancer) in 2007.

Too bad a drug to help break my nicotine addiction was not available when I was 20 years old. Richard Nixon's "War on Cancer" was just beginning when I took up cigarettes and became addicted. That "war" has been on-going for 40 years. It started out with the goal of defeating lung cancer, but in the intervening years the focus of cancer research turned to AIDS, breast cancer, and other forms of cancer. Lung cancer has languished without much progress or funding.

Ralph DeVito, the CEO of the American Cancer Society, Florida Division, tells me that the ACS has invested more than $3.2 billion in cancer research since 1946, of which $190 million has been specifically directed to lung cancer. What bothers me is that number is just 5 percent of all the money spent by the ACS on cancer research since 1946. It is a piddling amount when you consider the ACS raises nearly one billion dollars per year, Lung cancer accounts for 30 percent of all cancer deaths so shouldn't the research dollars devoted to lung cancer be higher than just five percent? Give me a break. ACS spends more money on executive pay than it does on lung cancer research.

The American Cancer Society's "solution" to the lung cancer epidemic has been to urge people to quit smoking, rather than invest in research. Anti-smoking campaigns have resulted in lung cancer becoming stigmatized as a "smoker's disease" in the same way AIDS was once considered the "lifestyle" disease of gays. And while it is true that not smoking will LOWER your risk of developing lung cancer that is NOT to say you are out of the woods, even if you quit DECADES ago.

Thanks to tens of billions of dollars in research funding, the annual death toll from AIDS has been reduced to 17,000 people a year in the U.S. AIDS is now a chronic disease that can be held at bay and successfully treated. Without enormous research funding, the death toll in the U.S. from AIDS would undoubtedly be much higher.

Similarly, the five-year survival rate for breast cancer has increased to 89 percent from 75 percent and the annual death rate from breast cancer is just under 40,000 people per year. Next to AIDS, breast cancer has received the greatest amount of federal cancer research funding. In fact, the enormous success of breast cancer advocates in raising awareness and funding has resulted in people believing that breast cancer is the No. 1 cancer killer in women. It's not....not even close.

Lung cancer kills 160,000 people per year. More than 220,000 new cases are diagnosed each year. Lung cancer is on the rise in women, who began openly smoking since the 1960's. (Remember the alluring Virginia Slims TV ads of that era that said "You've Come a Long Way Baby"?) Lung cancer use to be a primarily male disease. Now it kills 80,000 women a year, twice as many women as breast cancer, and three times as many men as prostate cancer. You sure have come a long way, baby. Be careful what you wish for!

I guess you could say that I got what I deserve for smoking all those years. Of course, I now regret the day I had my first cigarette, the way an alcoholic regrets his first drink.

Does the fact that I smoked mean I deserve to get cancer? Who is asking the question of why just 15 percent of all smokers get lung cancer (and 85 percent of smokers do not)? Is there a genetic predisposition to developing lung cancer? Research might answer these questions.

Today there are 70 million Americans like me who quit smoking. About 15 percent of us — one in six — will develop lung cancer one day. That's 14 million people who will die within five years of their diagnosis if things don't change. And what about people who never smoked? Did you realize they account for 10-15 percent of lung cancer patients? That's 20,000 — 30,000 people each year whose life will be cut short who didn't smoke a day in their life. Don't they deserve a little consideration?

Let's get real. As long as we are going to blame smokers for lung cancer, we should at least concede that more should have been done over the past 40 years. Shouldn't there be a method for screening people who smoked by now? Why hasn't the $8 billion a year in federal taxes collected from cigarette sales at least be earmarked for lung cancer research? Don't the people who pay tobacco taxes deserve to benefit something from those dollars?

Lung cancer is one of the deadliest forms of cancer because it is rarely detected early. There are no nerve endings in your lung, so tumors can grow without pain or discomfort. By the time there are symptoms, like a persistent cough, it is usually too late. Lung cancer's five-year survival rate (from date of diagnosis to death) is just 16 percent. The survival rate for late stage disease (Stage III and IV, which is most cases) is just 5 percent. I'm a Stage III survivor and just lucky to be alive today.

Lung cancer has been and remains the No. 1 cancer killer, taking more lives each year than breast, colon, prostate, kidney and melanoma COMBINED. Lung cancer accounts for a full 30 percent of ALL cancers deaths. The survival rate for lung cancer has hardly changed since the war on cancer began in 1971 yet there are fewer research dollars devoted to lung cancer than any other major cancer group.

People typically don't survive lung cancer, so lung cancer does not have a voice. We don't have a sea of survivor advocates. The fact is lung cancer is not the national research priority that it should be. Someone needs to speak up for the millions of people yet to be diagnosed. As a very rare lung cancer survivor, I feel that duty falls to me.

Epilogue —
A Second Chance at Life

In October of 2007 I went for my annual physical complaining of a cough. I thought it might be allergies — maybe mold in the new office. My doctor ordered an X-ray. The next day he called me in to the office to give me the bad news. In plain view on the X-ray he showed me a gigantic, baseball-sized tumor in the upper posterior of my right lung. He ordered a CT-guided needle biopsy for the next day. That is how my cancer journey began. I went home in shock not knowing what to do next or who to tell.

The biopsy confirmed that I had locally advanced non-small cell lung cancer. Based on size and other factors, my cancer was Stage IIIA. Because the tumor was intertwined with my central chest, it was inoperable. The only treatment available to me was radiation and chemotherapy. After the initial meeting with my oncologist, I thought I was a walking dead man.

The first thing Yoko and I did was put my affairs in order. I wanted to make sure she would be OK without me. I created a trust so that if she remarried, my assets would pass to our three daughters. I created an agreement with my business partner to sell my business in installments so Yoko would have a few more years of income. The silver lining of a cancer diagnosis, I thought, was having plenty of time to prepare to die.

I remember being sad that I would not be around to see my daughters with their own families. Worst of all, I was not going to have time to leave them any legacy to remember me by. I began to focus on the fact that in a single generation, my very existence would be forgotten. My grandchildren will never know me or remember me.

I began writing a blog to share my last thoughts and feelings with my daughters and to leave some sort of written account of my existence. My writings were emotional ramblings that documented my day to day thoughts as I went through nearly a year of treatments.

A written account of my life was one way for me to leave a legacy. Another would be to leave something of value to be handed down from one generation to the next. I decided to purchase artwork that, in time, might grow in value. I thought that art, over a few generations, could become a part of our family history. It would be a way to be remembered.

I did not tell anyone, other than my immediate family, about my cancer diagnosis. I am a financial advisor and I did not want people knowing that I have a life expectancy shorter than one market cycle. I was afraid that my clients might leave me or that I might never get a new client. Neither of these fears materialized.

In the end, blogging was how people learned about my diagnosis. I quickly discovered the sheer impossibility of keeping a secret in a small town. So I decided (like George Costanza in "Seinfeld") to "do the opposite" and go public. I am glad to say that no client ever fired me because I have cancer and I now make a habit of telling potential new clients about my disease before they decide to engage me.

After an initial eight weeks of treatment, my doctor told me that was all "evidence-based medicine" could do for me. We knew that the tumor had shrunk significantly, but it was not gone entirely. Billions of cancer cells were still roaming around in my body. I was not comforted to know that there was nothing more medical science could do.

I elected to have a second round of chemo to treat the cancer in my body "systemically." The idea was to kill any remaining cancer cells and prevent metastatic disease. That second round of chemo continued for 16 weeks. Again, there was "no evidence" that having a second round of chemo for someone with Stage III inoperable lung cancer was a good idea. I figured I had nothing to lose.

Oddly, lung cancer patients rarely die from lung disease. They typically die from metastatic disease to the bones or brain or some other vital organ. That is what eventually killed my mother-in-law, who died from metastatic lung cancer to the bones and brain.

I learned that the second round of chemo I had undertaken would treat cancer cells in my body, but not cancer cells that may be lingering in my brain. The "blood-brain" barrier prevents chemo from reaching the brain.

I was more worried about being disabled than dying. If I died, my family would be fine. If I was disabled with a brain tumor, I might drag them all down with me. Again, there was no evidence that brain radiation works as a preventative for someone like me, but then, there is no evidence that it doesn't work either.

After I walked my oldest daughter down the aisle in June 2008, I elected to have whole brain radiation treatment as a preventative. I struggled with the decision to do this, since, once again, there was "no evidence" it would help. In the end, I figured I would regret not doing it if I developed a brain tumor. Now, at least, if a brain tumor develops, at least I can be satisfied that I did all I could to prevent it.

After going through brain radiation, I found a Stage III clinical trial for a drug called Stimuvax, a vaccine intended to boost the immune system to fight cancer. I was lucky enough to be eligible to enroll in the trial and began a series of shots beginning in the fall of 2008. I am still getting shots, which requires my driving to an oncologist in New Port Richey every six weeks.

The trial I have enrolled in is a double blind study. Two thirds of the 1,200 enrolled patients are getting Stimuvax and one third get a placebo. Neither my doctor nor I know if I am getting the drug or a placebo.

October 2011 marks the fourth anniversary since my diagnosis. Believe it or not, these have been some of the best years of my life. I have doubled my business, creating greater security for my family, I've helped launch the Virginia B Andes Community Clinic, I've formed the Florida Chapter of the National Lung Cancer Partnership and organized the SW Florida Free to Breathe to raise lung cancer awareness and funding, I've written more than

140,000 words about my life and my battle with cancer, I've witnessed my youngest daughter graduate from college and my oldest daughter becoming a mother.

For me, cancer has made me focus on the things that are really important in life. I am a different person since I was diagnosed four years ago, and I am trying to make each and every day count. I hope the things I am doing now will create a lasting legacy.

Acknowledgements

As much as I enjoy writing and expressing my thoughts in words, I never thought I would have the time to write a book for publication. Writing a book has been a life ambition that I never expected to complete, especially after being diagnosed with lung cancer. This book is most certainly not "War and Peace" but thanks to lung cancer, I finally had the motivation to get busy and start writing! Death is as hard a deadline as you get.

When I began, I was blogging purely for emotional therapy. That morphed into keeping my family and friends informed about my health. They were the ones who liked what I was writing and encouraged me to continue, so they are the ones to be thanked (or blamed) for this book, which is the end result of their egging me on.

Once my private family blogs were public, I thought that lung cancer patients might benefit from what I had to say about living with cancer. (When I started, I was expecting to write about what is like to die from lung cancer! I'll save that ending for another book…sometime in the very distant future.)

After nearly a year of blogging, I approached the Charlotte Sun, my local newspaper, to see if it would have an interest in printing a weekly column called "Living with Cancer." I met with Jennifer Wadsworth, the editor of the Sun's Feeling Fit magazine at the time, who had just lost her mother to lung cancer. I did not have to do a lot of arm twisting before Jennifer enthusiastically agreed to begin publishing my column. What a God Wink!

I will forever be grateful to Jennifer and the Sun Newspapers for supporting me and my effort to shine a light on lung cancer over the past three years. Many thanks to fellow Rotarian Dave Powell, the publisher of Feeling Fit, and Karin Lillis, Feeling Fit's current editor, for their continued support for raising lung cancer awareness. I'm grateful for the generosity of the Sun Newspapers in sponsoring the Southwest Florida Free to Breathe 5K Run/Walk and One Mile Memorial Walk and helping me promote this local event to benefit lung cancer research.

Of course, I must thank my team of Florida doctors and specialists for helping me survive lung cancer long enough to be able to write a book. In particular I have to thank Dr. Scott Lunin and the nurses at Florida Cancer Specialists in Port Charlotte, Dr. David Rice and the nurses and technicians at 21st Century Oncology in Port Charlotte, Dr. Lary Robinson at Moffitt Cancer Center in Tampa, Dr. John Rioux at Fawcett Memorial Hospital in Port Charlotte, Dr. Thomas Fabian at Advanced Imaging and Dr. James White at Harbor Imaging also in Port Charlotte, my "study doctor" Dr. K.S. Kumar, Kim Graves, Sissi Hethershaw and the nurses at Cancer Care Centers of Florida in New Port Richey, and Dr. George Nackley at Millennium Physicians Group, who back in 2007 discovered my lung cancer just in the nick of time. I also want to thanks Dr Antoine Dakouny who now quarterbacks my large team of doctors. I would not be here in good health without all of you.

There are many other people to thank for the support and encouragement they have provided to me and my family. My Rotary friends are among my best friends, and within that special clutch of people I have to thank my golfing buddy Chris Maher, who just makes life fun, another golfing buddy, Kirby Rowe, who serves as Chris's straight man and is simply a kind-hearted gentleman, club comedian Len Johnson and his wife Dori, who have been faithful readers of my column, and Don Gasgarth, the owner of Charlotte County Ford, who has been a tremendous financial supporter and sponsor of the Free to Breathe 5K event in Southwest Florida. Special thanks also go to my very dear friends Brian and Lori Brunderman, who treat Yoko and me like we are family and are always giving to others.

I have to also thank my life-long friend and junior high school track rival, Eric Madsen, who called me regularly during my illness, prayed for me, and not infrequently corrected my spelling. Eric inspired me to write. I only wish I was as good a writer as he is. Luckily…I am faster.

I want to thank my friends Geof and Mary Grace Lorah, with whom I have a special connection. Mary Grace lost her sister to lung cancer. Mary's sister was the same age as me and was diagnosed with the same disease as me at nearly the same time as me, but she departed this world within six months of her diagnosis. I often think about that and wonder why she is now gone and I have been spared. I want Geof and Mary to know that I think about Mary's sister quite often. She and others who lost their battle with lung cancer are the inspiration for my advocating for lung cancer research and funding. Thank you for all you have done to help.

I need to say something to my good friend and spiritual mentor, Janet Minerich. Thank you, Janet, for putting me on your prayer list and inviting Yoko and me to your God Wink group. Our discussions of faith and religion have been uplifting. I know prayers are why I am still here and I know God holds a special place in his heart for you. The same goes for lung cancer survivor Irene Gargiulo and her husband Carlo, who work with me advocating for lung cancer, organize and run Charlotte County's lung cancer support group, and pray fervently for everyone they know with lung cancer. Their faith in God is inspiring.

I have to thank Dr. Joan Schiller, President, Dr. Regina Vidivar, Executive Director, and the staff of the National Lung Cancer Partnership for their leadership in helping to bring awareness, hope and change to the issue of lung cancer. Working together I know we are going to make a difference. Thank you for your dedication to our cause.

Finally I want to thank my family, especially my mother, Ann, my sisters, Jane, Linda and Peggy, my brother Frank and their spouses and children. Even though I don't see you often, you are always in my heart. I am grateful to you for your enduring love and prayers.

Life would not be worth living without the unconditional love of my wife, Yoko, and my girls, Paula, June and Jessie, and our growing family. Thank you for inspiring me every day to keep on living. I want to see what comes next. Nothing in this world gives me greater joy and happiness than you.

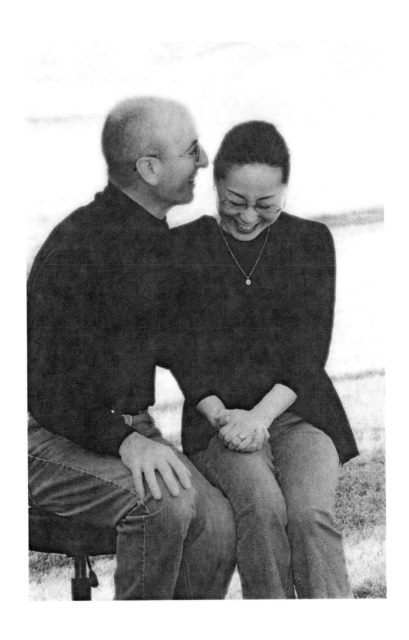